D0324261

RB
27
.G66
*1985

Gonzalez-Crussi, F.
    Notes of an
anatomist

LIBRARY/LRC
OUACHITA TECHNICAL COLLEGE
P.O. BOX 816
MALVERN, ARKANSAS 72104

NOTES OF AN ANATOMIST

OUACHITA TECHNICAL COLLEGE

NOTES
OF AN
ANATOMIST

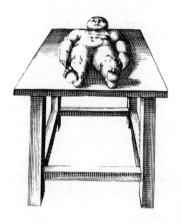

F. Gonzalez-Crussi

HARCOURT BRACE JOVANOVICH, PUBLISHERS

San Diego   *New York*   *London*

OUACHITA TECHNICAL COLLEGE

HBJ

Copyright © 1985, 1984 by F. Gonzalez Crussi, M.D.

All rights reserved. No part of this publication may be reproduced or transmitted in any form or by any means, electronic or mechanical, including photocopy, recording, or any information storage and retrieval system, without permission in writing from the publisher.

Requests for permission to make copies of any part of the work should be mailed to:
Permissions, Harcourt Brace Jovanovich, Publishers, Orlando, Florida 32887.

Excerpts from "Reflections on Child Abuse" appeared in *The Child's Doctor* 1 (Fall 1984) (the journal of the Children's Memorial Hospital of Chicago, Ill.) by special permission.

Library of Congress Cataloging in Publication Data

Gonzalez-Crussi, F.
  Notes of an anatomist.

  1. Anatomy, Pathological—Miscellanea.   2. Abnormalities, Human—Miscellanea.   I. Title.
RB27.G66 1985   616.07   85–776
ISBN 0–15–167285–7

Designed by Joy Taylor

Printed in the United States of America
First Edition

  B C D E

RB
27
.G66
1985

To my wife, Wei, whose help made this possible

CONTENTS

On Embalming   1

Twins   14

Unpeaceful Afterlife   24

Of Some Bodily Appendages   36

Myasis   44

The Body from Outside
(With Notes on the Outside of the Inside)   51

The Dead as a Living   62

Reflections on Child Abuse   72

Teratology   91

On Male Genital Anatomy   110

Notes   131

NOTES OF AN ANATOMIST

ON EMBALMING

C EREMONY and ritual spring from our heart of hearts: those who govern us know it well, for they would sooner deny us bread than dare alter the observance of tradition. And yet funeral ceremonies can change. The Dayak people of Borneo used to preserve the body of a dead chief in the communal house of the living, a practice they had to abandon under the pressure of Dutch officials who did not take kindly to this form of mixed company. With equally commendable sanitary zeal, authorities in India have been known to oppose the ancient customs of the Parsis of Bombay, Zoroastrian votaries, who place the bodies of their dead atop circular constructions, where, in a matter of hours, vultures dispose neatly of all the fleshy parts. Europeans generally perceived a lurid aura about this ritual and showed little sympathy for what they saw as a "secret cult of death." Yet the Parsi custom dates its origins at least six centuries before the birth of Christ and was inspired by the currently much-vaunted goal of decreasing ecologic contamination: the Zoroastrian believes the dead body so unclean that it would contaminate the "pure elements" of the universe—earth, fire, and water.

In Europe and the United States embalming was practically unknown before the latter part of the eighteenth century. The modern technic of this procedure is generally attributed to the Scottish anatomist William Hunter. Before his day, and in the United States up to the years of the Civil War, cadavers that had to be transported or kept unburied for days were simply packed in ice. There were "cooling boards," concave devices filled with ice in which the body could fit snugly, but, beyond this rudimentary inventiveness, it may be said that corpse technology had not really been put at the service of the common people.

Consider this telling difference between East and West: among the ancient Egyptians, embalming was but one aspect of a life oversaturated with things spiritual and preoccupied with the possible fate of the soul after the body had perished. In the industrial West, there has been an equally universal and all-encompassing preoccupation. It is called desire for profit, and, as will become apparent here, it has done much for the spread of the practice of embalming.

In the West, embalming and greed seem to have been wedded from the beginning. John Hunter, younger brother of the Scottish anatomist, came across an exceptional opportunity to apply his brother's methods. A wealthy woman, Mrs. Martin Van Butchell, under motives obscure and indecipherable, wrote a peculiar will. It was her intention, duly legalized by seals and signatures, that her surviving husband should have control of her fortune only for as long as she would remain above ground. Upon her demise, her husband acted with a determination all the more admirable for being mixed with grief. John Hunter was summoned to the homestead. Mrs. Van Butchell's remains were injected intra-arterially with fluids of recent invention, and the lady ended up, fashionably clad in her best finery, inside a glass-lidded container, before which she received friends and relatives.

After these auspicious beginnings, the career of the embalming practice made impressive gains, but nowhere as sound as in the United States, where the government threw its full weight behind it. Here, embalming became mandatory by law whenever the interval between death and burial exceeds forty-eight hours (twenty-four in some states) or when the body must be transported a certain distance. To say that embalming is big business in America would be, as everyone knows, a great understatement. According to recent statistics, less then 8 percent of the lifeless population of this country is disposed of by cremation, and since alternative methods of disposal, such as cannibalism or Zoroastrian exposure, must be very infrequently practiced in America, it follows that embalming continues to be an economically important activity. This is true from the standpoint of the total economy of the nation as well as from the more restricted viewpoint of individual enterprise.

However spurious or suspect the origins of Western embalming, the pathologist ought to acknowledge his gratitude to the practitioners of this trade. Theirs is an activity that cannot be dismissed as menial, in spite of its frequent unpleasantness. At its most perfected and professional, it is no exaggeration to say that it should be called an art. Without the skillful intervention of dieners, funeral house directors, and morgue attendants, the pathologist's task would be much more onerous and frequently impossible, for it is part of his job to secure bodily parts for conscientious study—in some cases entire mandibles, eyes, femurs, or vertebral columns.

On a rare occasion, the pathologist, at the completion of his task, has looked back on the remains lying on the table and felt a chill upon realizing that professional zeal has caused him to alter the human form in a manner apt to be called a defilement. The dead possess an identity, granted by the living through the agency of intact form; so long as form remains, a cadaver remains "the same one" for associates and relatives, for friend and foe. But without spine or limbs or eyes (which virtually never are removed during an autopsy study), the form is altered and diminished; without ribs, the dead person is a frail manikin; without jaw, the human face is a grotesque mask. For the body to be viewed at this time by the most generous purveyors of identity, his loved ones, could mean disaster. Such catastrophic events are, happily, almost unheard of. In the exceptional case of removal of a large bodily part, the adroit ministrations of the mortician will avert a sad outcome. In place of absent bones he places rigid rods or sticks; he restores and reconstructs, closes off incisions, and fills up gaps. In the end, like a proud craftsman, he sits back and contemplates his finished production awaiting the final verdict: the "viewing" ceremony. And since the dead are often the worn-out, shattered rejects of life, he can aspire, like a true artist, to improve the work of nature. Cotton pledgets under the eyelids will counteract the effects of dehydration; placed inside the cheeks, they will make the hollowed-out appearance of consumption yield to a more robust semblance of life. The eyes, fixed in a dilated stare of horror, are carefully closed according to the *Manual of the Embalmer* "so that the upper eyelid covers exactly two-thirds of the globe"; then they are smeared with Vaseline to prevent drying. And even the pallor of extreme anemia (the color of shrouds) or advanced jaundice (yellow as gamboge) will disappear under the influence of dyes and bleaching agents mixed in the embalming fluid, distributed under brand names like Blossom and Spring and promoted with catchy slogans in morticians' magazines that read: "As if he were sleeping" or "Bring back the colors of spring." Yes; as long as the somewhat macabre custom of deathwatch endures, the pathologist will need beside him those dexterous assistants whose calling means protection from charges that range between minor fluke and hideous sacrilege.

When younger, I cherished the romantic notion that

in the age of the New Kingdom of Egypt secrets of embalming were discovered that surpassed in effectiveness the most advanced technics of our day. The image of priests and mortician-priests uttering magical incantations inside pharaonic tombs and preserving dead bodies from decomposition for two thousand years is sure to fire the romantic fantasy of any youth. It was with some disappointment that I learned that, in terms of sheer technical efficacy, the ancient Egyptians achieved only mediocre results and that their methods are neither mysterious nor unexplainable to us. Apparently, the Egyptians covered the dead with blocks of natre, or natron, a natural salt found in the Nile Valley. Instead of being an esoteric formula, natron turns out to be a mixture of rather commonplace chemicals, namely, sodium carbonate and sodium bicarbonate, with a varying amount of impurities, chiefly sodium sulfate and common salt. Thus the Egyptians merely "salted" their corpses, slowly extracting water, which is indispensable for the enzymatic actions that account for decomposition; at the same time, the salts produced a weak fixation.

The desired effects were more easily achieved by removal of the viscera, which were placed in canopic jars, but the process was slow; a job was not completed in less than a month or two. And at the end of this lengthy preparation, the task was not over for these forebears of the modern embalmer. Followed the laborious swathing with bandages soaked in resins and gum resins and the sprinkling with scents, all of which are now known to possess antibacterial agents. All according to elaborate ritual: the bandage of Nekheb on the well-oiled forehead; the bandage of Hathor on the face; and there was also the gilding of the nails, and the crystal to lighten the face, and carnelian to strengthen the steps of the deceased in the underworld. There followed a strange ceremony that stands in curious opposition to ours. This was called "the opening of the mouth." Mouth and eyes of the recently embalmed cadaver, or its effigy, were pried open by means of specially designed instruments held by a priest, in contrast to our "pious" gesture of closing the same natural orifices in the recently departed. The very concrete ideas of the Egyptians about the voyage awaiting the dead might explain this singular gesture: the deceased had to be in fit condition to pronounce the sacred incantations that were passwords to the beyond. Think of the responsibility of these ancestors of the profession: careless facial bandaging meant considerably more than a pardonable fluke; it meant precluding an immortal soul from gaining salvation, by gagging!

Though divested of their mystery, the ministrations of these predecessors of present-day morticians remain admirable. How many craftsmen, or even renowned artists, today can feel confident that their work will be admired two thousand years hence, as we admire the excellent state of preservation of Seti I? This is not to say that all Egyptian embalmers were equally competent. Archeologists must be uniquely aware that there were bunglers, especially at those times when the suspense attending the undoing of bandages turns to dismay upon discovering, instead of the majestic presence of a ruler come down the ages in gold and lapis lazuli, a heap of crumbling filth swarming with insects. Still, the Egyptian technic was compatible with a respectful and solemn attitude toward the dead. On the authority of a distinguished pathologist, Guido Majno, we know that they neither immersed them in brine, as they did—and we do—with fish, nor roasted them over slow fires, as some South American Indians have been known to do—and as we are wont to do with chickens, producing comparable results. Their procedure was, in the graphic saying of Majno, "mothballing, and with weak mothballs at that."[1]

What is apparent to the modern embalmer, in stark contrast with the ancient calling, is that all these carryings-on are strictly for the benefit of the living. The questions are seriously raised among the practitioners of the trade whether the remains should be "laid out" with glasses on, whether cosmetics should be applied, and whether the placement of dentures is indispensable. Not for a minute is it assumed that the decedent will need to have his vision corrected or his denture fit for biting an apple; nor is he in need of any of the three shades of pink cosmetic distributed by B. and G. Products, guaranteed to reproduce "nature's own skin texture . . . the velvety appearance of living tissue." Among the highest spheres of power in the National Funeral Directors Association, the statement that embalming is a procedure designed with the living in mind would not be received without controversy. It is difficult, however, to agree on just how embalming benefits the living. For reasons not hard to guess, officialdom within the NFDA proclaims that an open-coffin ceremony serves laudable purposes, to wit, aiding in the direct expression of grief, providing a suitable atmosphere for mourning, and helping the bereaved to face the finality of death. The problem is one that has been much pondered, without a single answer yet in sight. It is counterargued that the display of the body may be traumatic to certain individuals, especially to children, even when forewarned and instructed on what to expect; that "viewing" is hardly an aid to contemplate death when the "viewee" has been meticulously restored to impart to its external appearance a close semblance of life; that a person's ability to grasp the concept of death is the product of his total life experience, quite independent of "viewing"; and that, in any case, a memorial service is sufficient reminder of the ineluctability of death, thus rendering immaterial the open or closed state of the coffin's lid.

I believe there is at the core of the embalmer's officiousness a desire to remove the harrowing aspects of death, to expunge its painful appearance, and to erase all hurtful experiences for the survivors. I also believe that this is not altogether contemptible. Perhaps this desire to beautify the unavoidable miseries of an essentially finite, hence decaying, existence is a conspicuous feature of the American way of life. At least, such a thesis was proposed and developed by the French philosopher Jacques Maritain, who illustrated it with the following autobiographical anecdote.

Maritain, newly arrived in the United States, was entirely taken by the general civility and democratic warmth which he, like most foreigners, noticed immediately upon arrival. In academic circles, he observed, the students are not treated arrogantly by their professors but consort amicably with them; and the latter, regardless of their rank, see it as their duty to ease the way of learning for the students. This contrasts with the rigid scholastic mores and the unbridgeable chasm that often separates, in other countries, the humble student from the haughty pinnacles of professional arrogance. In public offices, transactions are closed expeditiously and, allowing for the inherently frustrating nature of red tape, with considerably less humiliation than attend dealings with the bureaucracy in other lands. This polite efficiency he found also in his visits to the dentist. Immaculately attired nurses and dental assistants, working in a spotless environment among gleaming equipment, directed him, positioned him, inquired of his needs, and prepared him for the reparative dental work. All was done with the utmost efficiency and with no other interruptions than required by brief, polite questions: "Are you comfortable?" "Is everything all right?"

Suddenly, while sitting in the dentist's chair, the thought came to him that if he were to suffer a fatal heart attack right then, all these professionals, technicians, assistants, and attendants would continue to perform their most attentive, purposeful, and determined services. A cold sweat covered his forehead as he imagined the smiling nurses, professional composure undaunted, laying him out on a bier. Everything would be as orderly, methodical, and efficient as before: his arms would be brought together so that his hands would touch each other in a pious and collected gesture; his body would be smoothly transferred into a well-designed coffin with chromed edges; and all expert finishing touches would be put on his remains by attendants whose unruffled expressions would be the same as when, minutes before, they inquired of him: "Are you comfortable?" and "Is everything all right?" This vision so shockingly conflicted with Maritain's conception of a Catholic passing away to await the Day of Resurrection that he became the first patient ever to change dentists for entirely theological reasons.

Maritian was highly partial to the whitewashing instinct of white Anglo-Saxon America. In this he saw neither insensitivity nor hypocrisy. He believed in an inherent "goodness" of the American people that leads them to attempt to efface all the potentially hurtful aspects of life. Misery and suffering seem, upon but slight reflection, the inescapable lot of life; even more so: part and parcel of life, like breathing. Through a kind of heroic contumaciousness, Americans are impelled to disbelieve this appalling truth. On the positive side, this monumentally wistful attitude forms the basis of their superior technological ingenuity. If life appears to many as a fatal stupefying bondage of sweat and toil, Americans will counter by inventing machines and gadgets to shake the yoke— the same gadgets that, incidentally, will be avidly taken up by those very critics who thunder against the "dehumanizing" perils of American technology. When the funeral customs of Americans are examined by this light, it is not easy to be overly critical of the ceremony of "viewing" an embalmed dead person. Death, like the sun, cannot be viewed directly; it is like an unfathomable void that gives us a sort of metaphysical vertigo if we so much as go near the edge of the cliff. Yet if there is an element of the ridiculous in a custom that substitutes a "restored" corpse, made up to look like a living doll, for the uncontemplable spectacle of death, we must confess that the same is true for most symbolic ritual. And then all harsh criticism recedes in front of the discovery that this is yet another attempt, however naive, of a people bent on removing all unpleasantness from life; a further manifestation of the American's "goodness" that wills universal politeness and whose motto might well be "Cleanliness and contentment for all!"

The ridiculous, however, is the least of dangers in such an attitude. Behind the illusion that life can be a succession of smiling scenes, with neither pain nor passion, lurks the delusion that death without anguish can be bought for money in an over-the-counter transaction. Cash, check, or credit card. And behind this counter hides the ugly mien of philistinism, for which it is impossible to feel much sympathy. In the *Consumers Report on Conventional Funerals and Burial* there is an account of alarming excesses of commercialism that plague these services. In one case, mourners were introduced into a richly furnished antechamber in which each piece of decor represented, one may reasonably suppose, an extra charge on the bill: flowers at so many dollars; background organ music for such a price; and so on.[2] After a while an usher announced that Mrs. X was ready to receive the visitors, and the mourners went, treading on thick carpets between floral arrangements and parting dark draperies, into another room of still more luxurious decor that seemed right out of *faux* Versailles. There, as if she were a duchess, or at least a countess in a second-rate Hollywood motion picture, sat Mrs. X, or rather the remains of Mrs. X, on a canopied bed abundant in lace and ribbons, dressed in a silk robe and propped up by cushions. Mark what private enterprise can do: the death ceremony transformed into a social visit, with a touch of vulgarity proportionate to the size of the payer's pocket! In another case, a Louisiana entrepreneur hit upon the felicitous idea of organizing the "viewing" ceremony around the "drive-in" concept. Mourners could look from the reassuring security of their automobiles into a display room where the decedent was aptly shown in a most collected and well-kept attitude behind a glass window, reposing on a bier whose end was surmounted by a cross framed with blue neon-gas light tubes. While under interrogation by the congressional committee on irregular funeral practices, the businessman defended well his unorthodox services: families could mourn and pay their visit at all hours, without leaving the soothing enclosure of their own automobiles; they did not have to pay any attention to details of their dress or worry about being the targets of gossip, thus being free to express their grief in a wholesome way; and, once their visit was over, they could simply lower the window of their car, sign a thick register book within arm's reach, and "drive on."

Whereas such practices seem to step on the toes of our sense of righteousness, we might do well, before voicing our indignant execration, to probe the public sentiment on the matter. In letters to the syndicated columnist Ann Landers, complaints were expressed on the charging methods of funeral directors. In particular, severe reproof went to those who sell expensive garments with which to dress the cadaver. It was thought that luxurious raiment, difficult to justify for the living, is assuredly a wanton waste on the dead. The expensive clothes are often sold because some undertakers prepare photographs (and oil paintings!) of the decedent, which are later sold to the relatives who, grief stricken, are often vulnerable to these swindles. With her proverbial impartiality, the columnist also published letters of persons who took a different view of the subject. Among these, there was a widow who wrote, "I wouldn't take a million dollars for the pictures I made of my husband laid out in his new blue suit. He looked better in that box than he had any time in the last ten years."

As a pathologist who has seen no rise in his life insurance policy premiums despite customary corpse handling, I am naturally skeptical of reports that extoll embalming as a public health blessing. Lack of embalming of cadavers does not seem a cause of devastating epidemics in most countries, and most countries fail to routinely practice this procedure. For the fact that epidemics are uncommon we ought to acknowledge a greater debt to sanitation engineers or public health officials then to embalmers. Bacteria do proliferate in a cadaver, as anyone can confirm who is of sound nose and comes within fifty paces of the autopsy room. Highly pathogenic organisms proliferate too, but elementary precautions of antisepsis, like the wearing of surgical mask and gloves,seem to adequately protect all exposed personnel. Morgue-acquired infections are part of the romance and lore of the autopsy suite, but one hears of the macabre saga mostly secondhand. I have not been impressed by either the frequency or the nefarious quality of infections therein contracted by persons who live there day by day, although the specialized literature mentions individual instances of dire diseases acquired in this environment.

The practice of embalming dead American citizens is so massively successful that, as is well known, a person living in the United States is statistically likelier to live closer to a funeral home than to a police station or a fire department building. This comes from profit consciousness, not from enlightened legislation. The funeral industry is so well organized and so expertly directed that its revenues are unlikely to decrease, even if funeral customs were to change. Should cremation become the most popular form of disposal of remains, private enterprise will prove equal to the challenge and will be ready to diversify, as they say in financial circles, and to control. However, as a pathologist, too, I am not ready to condemn the practice of embalming as a shameless farce or to pass it up as nothing but a sordid hoax played by the greedy on the gullible. Rather, I see in it an impulse, not without nobility, to prevent, or at least decelerate, the ruin of the human body. Commercialism and dishonesty aside, the embalmer obeys that obscure dictate that would have us stave off, or at least retard, the decay of this marvel. It is our primeval vigor, our deepest creative prepotency, our basic fund of antideath energy, that infuses us with the wish, however irrational, to make the corruptible undecaying and the impermanent eternal. The ancients fancied that the soul did not abandon the body on a sudden but even after death it lingered on for forty-two days, departing gradually and as if by stages. Da Vinci reflected on this theme and thought that it was quite fitting that the soul should dally, for the body is so wondrous a habitation that the soul could not find it easy to part with it, and finding it so painful to quit its mortal domicile, it hesitates. Later, that delicately spiritual writer Paul Valéry, on reading the autobiographical passage of Leonardo that contains these reflections, was greatly intrigued. This was for Valéry a metaphysical system of most peculiar originality: that the farewell scene between body and soul should be imagined as capable of "bringing tears to the eyes . . . of the soul"! Leonardo, it is very important to remember, had personally dissected scores of cadavers; his metaphysical construct may strike many as odd, but pathologists and embalmers should find it perfectly natural.

TWINS

I ndividual human life begins this way: The fertilized egg cell, even before it is implanted in the womb, transforms itself into a spherical mass of tightly packed cells, each of enormous potential but hardly different from its neighbors. There is nothing to suggest the human form, yet the germ of a human being is locked up inside. In our earliest beginnings, nature makes us perfect, for the sphere is the ideal receptacle of perfection. The perfect being, independent of externals and utterly self-sustaining, said Plato, ought to be like the sphere of the cosmos. Horace, musing over the unattainable ideal, described the wise man free from fear and master of his passions "who in himself is a whole, smoothed and rounded, so that nothing from outside can rest on its polished surface, and against whom Fortune in her onset is ever maimed" (*Satires*, bk. 2, satire 7, ll. 86–88).

It seems preordained, however, that we should soon stray away from perfection. Soon there appears a streaklike ridge, or chine, over the surface of the embryonic cell mass, and henceforth we pass into the realm of symmetry: there shall be a central axis, and around this axis right- or left-sidedness. By virtue of a central divide, all organs can organize with reference to a plane, and it is fitting that the technical name

for this dividing ridge should be that of "organizer," for it
seems to inspire, inform, and direct future embryonic tissues
rather than stand as a passive landmark. But the mysterious
influences that direct these transformations, though miracu-
lously precise, are not infallible. Thus a spherical embryo may
be cleft into halves by one divider and then again, as if by
accident, in two more halves by another divider whose very
powers of organization, awesome in their complexity, continue to be exercised as if impelled by a blind design that
took no notice of the original mishap and continued on, un-
swervingly, of its own inertia. The result is that in the end,
where the birth of a human infant was expected, as is proper
and right for the human species, the emergence of the first
child is followed by another one that looks like its exact
replica; and, sometimes, this is followed by another one, and,
in some cases, by still more, so that human procreation, apparently designed for the nourishment and containment of
one individual per cycle, comes to resemble the animal litters,
wherein multiplicity is the rule.

Every gestation is fundamentally portentous, but one that
so abruptly does away with predictable events and issues in
two, or more, products leaves us dumbfounded. The "prim-
itive" mind is likely to think of it as an inauspicious calamity,
or a happy augur; either a demeaning of the species by maleficent demons, or the gratuity of generous gods who wish
us well and rejoice over our increment. This is why the folklore of nations is inconsistent and contradictory with respect
to multiple births. In parts of Europe twins are brought to
attend weddings, for their presence is considered propitiatory
of fertility, but in rural Bulgaria the wedding ceremony in-
cludes symbolic steps designed to stave off the possibility of
twin births. The ancient Assyrians thought that the birth of
twins was inauspicious for common people but a cause for
celebration if it occurred within the royal family. Among the

Ashanti of West Africa, on the contrary, twins were generally welcome, but they were smothered when, born in the royal family, they posed problems for the crown's succession. Throughout the world, it was never clear whether to celebrate or to mourn. All that was clear was the whimsical nature of the event; whether caused by a demon to be appeased or a god to be thanked, it could not be known. Nor did it matter, for against superhuman fickleness we were powerless. Against supernatural volubility, no strategy avails; exorcism or invocation, propitiatory rite or symbolic repulse, each ran a fifty-fifty chance of being successful.

If societies had cause to be bewildered, so did twins. During our childhood, we grasp the meaning of identity and diversity in the world and in our own persons. We suddenly realize our uniqueness. In our childish idleness we imagine the possibility that in a different country, perhaps on a different planet, there may be another being endowed with the same physical and mental attributes that pass, in our world, for exclusively our own. But what science-fiction writers have imagined, a mirror-image reality existing alongside our universe, is no flight of fancy for the twin: his cotwin strongly reminds him of the plausibility of this imaginary world of reciprocal imaging. The diagnosis of identical twinning, before the advent of more sensitive tests, relied precisely on its demonstration: if one twin has a birthmark on the right shoulder, the other bears it on the left; if one's right eye is slightly darker than the left, the opposite is true for his cotwin; right-handedness in one, left-handedness in the other. And the parallels extend beyond physical equivalence. On March 11, 1979, the *Chicago Tribune* reported on the reunion of twins who had been given up for adoption at birth, had been reared by separate families, and had lived apart for thirty-nine years. In spite of not having seen each other for nearly forty years, each had a first marriage with a woman named Linda; each had divorced; each named a son James Allan; each then married a woman named Betty. Their hobbies, mechanical lettering and carpentry, were the same; their favorite resort area for vacations was the same beach in the St. Petersburg area; their occupations were similar. The identical twin, like the identical triplet, or any identical multiple, gazes into the shattered mirror of his own individuality with a perplexity that is directly proportional to the number of his brethren.

Locke defined self as consciousness and said that the little finger, while comprehended under that consciousness, is as much part of the self as what is most so; and that if the little finger were to be cut off and carry with it this consciousness, "it is evident that the little finger would be the person, and self would have nothing to do with the rest of the body." But a twin sees an entire being, an autonomous thinking and feeling homologue, whose compound nature more strongly than a severed little finger represents to the mind that it, too, has consciousness. And since this being, outwardly the same person as he, shared his beginnings in time and space, thus fulfilling the requisites that logic demands of identity, he must experience the odd sensation that his consciousness is shared and his self cleft twice, thrice, or more. In a sense, one might say that the twin is "beside himself," and the connotation of being dazzled or confounded that is embodied in the expression is more telling of the problems of identity besetting twins than many a learned treatise. Mark Twain summed up the twin's dilemma with humor. With utterly serious air he told a journalist that he had been, at the time of his birth, one member of a twin pair. Tragedy, he said, struck his family when one of the twins, unattended in the bathtub, drowned. As the two brothers were identical, it was very difficult, even for the parents, to tell who had drowned and who had survived. This tragedy so moved him that later he delved into the circumstances of the accident. In his quest he came to examine the hospital records, by which he found that the physician described a birthmark on his brother's back. Now, since he, Mark Twain, knew of the existence of a birthmark on his own back, he was forced to conclude: "It is he who survived; I drowned."

To explain multiple births, biologists multiply hypotheses. Identical twins may arise when the fertilized egg cell fortuitously splits into two spheres because of desultory changes in the environment. By recognizing this random disruption of a delicate ecology, biology does no more than acknowledge the existence of the fickle demon, without surprising his hand in the act of trickery. Or perhaps the splitting of the primordial sphere is not the effect of chance but the result of a duplicating factor inherent in the father's sperm, carried into the egg cell, much like a distraught burglar would leave behind a personal object in the house he intended to loot. Alternatively, the duplicating impetus may not be extraneous to the egg cell but may reside there waiting only for the signal to make its presence felt. Or, yet, no extraneous factor is required, nor is a signal needed, but human duplication could arise from a deficiency of the conditions that preside over the formation of singletons, as an absence of restraining influences instead of a surplus of formative ones; in which case multiple conception would be thought of as an excess resulting from a want, but neither of the two would be explained. And from this baroque coiling of biological theories, we infer that the biologist, like the maker of myths, is dumbfounded. The swindling god keeps substituting the peas under his thimbles too swiftly for anyone to detect the cheat; and the biologist, like all others, wishing to expose the trickery, can only admire the contrivance.

Externally, the pathologist's approach seems somewhat different. As usual, he adjusts his focus on the exceptional, the pathologic. Through deviancy, he hopes for glimpses of the underlying order. Hence his interest in monstrosities, which he so carefully classifies. And if he is not at the same time an experimentalist, he will be wont to pronounce, *ut quum facta sunt* (after the fact has occurred), "the interpretation that verifies his conjectures," as Cicero scornfully said of seers and fortune-tellers. To him, twinning per se is not "pathologic enough." Double conception, after all, may be conducted in a normal atmosphere of shared harmony; but any form of intrauterine discord is sure to polarize the pathologist's attention. Such, for instance, the "twin-to-twin transfusion syndrome," a form of imbalance in which one twin's circulation empties into placental vessels that divert the blood to his cotwin. As a result, the "recipient" twin is born large, ruddy, and plethoric, while his brother, the "donor," if he manages to survive, emerges pale, anemic, and wasted. The pathology of twinning is largely the history of sibling rivalry before birth. If the feud dates back to the stage when each twin was close to the sphere, its effects may be profound. In their clash for the womb's territory one may encroach upon the other, or, in their precocious wrestling, they may fail to disjoin. In each case the consequence is two sibs more or less fused to each other. The birth of such children has always elicited sensational accounts, such as this graphic one by Montaigne:

> Under his nipples [this child] was taken by, and glued to, another infant, a headless one, whose back furrow seemed full but was otherwise intact, although one of his arms was shorter than the other, having been broken at birth. Thus, the union had taken place between the nipples and the navel. The navel of the imperfect one could not be seen, but one could see the rest of his abdomen. All that was not joined, like the arms, buttocks, thighs, and legs of the imperfect one, hung pendulous and swinging from the other one, reaching down to his mid-calf. The

nurse added that he urinated from the two places; also, the limbs of this other one were living and nourished, just as his own, except for being smaller and tiny. (*"D'un enfant monstrueux"*)

In all these examples, asymmetry is wrought by the violence of prenatal strife, and of two prospective equals one emerges victorious, the other dead, vanquished, or maimed. Brotherly union, for once, results in weakness. "Together we are weaker" is the conjoined twin's motto. Some say that this physical fusion has been advantageous, but their stories are simply incredible. Regnault, with all the respectability of a cleric, wrote that the hunting party that accompanied Louis XIV in the forest of Compiègne, captured a wild goat with two heads, which nonetheless pranced and grazed with all the vigor of its single-headed congeners. And across the Rhine, another king is said to have come across an even more admirable animal. A conjoined hare was so formed as to exhibit a double set of limbs and heads. The fusion, according to the chronicler, had taken place along the dorsal plane in such a way that when one set of legs was resting on the ground, the second set was lifted toward the sky. This "Double Hare of Germany" astounded its persecutors by being able to run for long distances without showing signs of fatigue. The reason, says the quaint account, was that through periodic rolling on the ground the ingenious hare managed to alternate the use of each set of limbs and was on each turn carried by limbs that had been previously resting!

Twin fusion is, of course, compatible with longevity. This we know by the stories, always engrossing, of conjoined twins: the Biddenden Maids, fused at the arms; the Hungarian Sisters, joined at the pelvis; the conjoined twins of Bohemia; and the most famous of all, the Siamese twins, "stuck" to each other by a bridge going from abdomen to abdomen.

Fusion was only partial and did not hamper the development of separate identities. Thus we hear that, of the Siamese twins, Chang was outspoken and Chen quiet; this one timid, that one arrogant. Forced to subordinate all their activities to the inalterable fact of their physical togetherness, they learned to coordinate their steps while walking and, having married, scrupulously respected for many years the convenant to spend three days in the house of each one's spouse, in alternation. All of which did not stop an altercation when, on a certain day, Chang wished to take a bath and Chen did not. There were witnesses to the shouting of insults, and it is reported that they came to blows, for apparently physical pain was experienced by each one individually, although, if one contracted an infection, fever was manifested by both.

Of the Hungarian sisters, joined at the pelvis, medical reports say that they had a common rectum, a single external genital area, but two wombs and two birth canals. These are the only conjoined twins ever to have conceived. In times of Victorian prudishness, the two sisters appeared in the emergency room of a hospital, A's abdomen swollen, B's flat. Questioned about their sexual history, A adamantly denied, and B consistently supported her, even if, in the graphic pun of their biographer, "she should have been in a position to know." After A was delivered of a healthy baby, there was plenty of sassy commentary, although not without troubling religiophilosophical undertones. Given the described anatomical arrangement, it was asked, should they have one or two husbands? In like manner friars of early Spanish America argued over whether the holy rites of the Catholic Church should be administered once or twice to a pair of dying conjoined twins. This problem was solved, in this case, by an autopsy that showed that the liver was the only shared organ. Now, the liver was never seriously thought in theological circles to be the site of residence of the soul; therefore the case was firmly settled in favor of duality. This may be said to be a little known instance of a contribution of pathology to Christian theology.

An even more difficult quandary was posed by abnormal twins born in Medina-Sidonia on February 29, 1793. The conceptus had two heads, two necks, and four upper extremities, but only two legs. Parturition was difficult, and one foot was delivered first. As it became clear that the infant would soon die, the baptism and last rites were administered to the part—the foot—of the expected singleton. Upon delivery of the entire body, the problem was stated thus: assuming the existence of two immortal souls, which of the two had been baptized? This was the problem presented to Father Feijoo, the learned Jesuit who was to earn a place of distinction in Spanish literature. Feijoo's answer was dressed up in the most rigorous logic. Firstly, the existence of the soul could not be denied. The site of residence of the soul was a matter of debate; contending parties favored either the heart or the brain. Now, since all major viscera were duplicated, there could be no doubt that two independent souls were involved. Secondly, everyone wished to believe that both had been baptized, because Christian piety moves us to feel sorry for those who are deprived of the sovereign benefit of baptism. However, our desires count for little in front of the heavenly tribunal, and charitable wishes cannot repair the damage that is done. The search for truth must take precedence over our wistful expectations. Thirdly, a priest who baptizes performs an act that extends to a subject previously apprehended by the understanding. The words used, *ego te bapitzo*, refer to a single individual. No willful act can be extended to any other subject than that apprehended by the mind preceding, or accompanying, the act of volition, according to the formula: *nihil volitum, quin praecognitum*. Now, the baptizing priest had no idea that the foot on which he sprinkled holy water was, in effect, shared by two separate souls. Therefore, his understanding apprehended a single one, and by a volitional act he performed a ceremony that confers regenerative grace upon a single individual. Therefore, he used the wrong formula. Therefore, the ceremony was invalid. Therefore, none was baptized.

There is yet one more step. The binomial becomes AA, the "monster" of perfect symmetry; some call it Janus, pathologists cranio-thoraco-pagus. Imagine two profiles meeting on a median plane of fusion, as if two lovers would have wished to fuse while they embraced and their wish had been granted. The foreheads are fused, the noses have blended. Viewed frontally, two eyes can be seen, although each one is actually in profile. And this strange face repeats itself in the back—or is it the front?—of Janus. The necks are fused into one, and so are the chest and abdomen. There are two hearts, but they are joined by a common aorta. Two mouths, but the intestines are shared. Human beings are supposed to have a front and a back, a top and a bottom. But when the front is also the back and the left is as much left as it is right, can we say that there is top and bottom? The duality of Janus is more than startling: it is impossible. Three centuries ago Sir Thomas Browne denied the existence of amphisbaena, the snake with a head at each end, on theoretical grounds, "for the senses being placed at both extreams doth make both ends anterior, which is impossible." But a pathologist, who has seen Janus, chimera, cyclops, acardius, and mermaid (sirenomelia), no longer doubts the existence of the impossible. Instead, he will concede the truth in this statement of Borges: "The zoology of dreams is far poorer than the zoology of the Maker."

UNPEACEFUL AFTERLIFE

L ORD BYRON thought that no more beautiful epitaph could be imagined than one he saw at the cemetery of La Certosa, in Bologna: "So-and-so *implora pace*." It is said that Alfred de Vigny even wished it inscribed on his own tomb. Peace, and nothing more. The ultimate reward: peace, the true and only good.

It must be owned, however, that there are men of dispositions much less calm than the likes of Byron and Vigny. When "peace on earth" is uttered, the salutation yet says: "to men of gentle will." Thus, peace is wished only on a very limited segment of humankind. And it is well that the gracious greeting should be exclusionary, for temper and character vary so much that one man's guerdon may well be the next man's punishment. Bellicose natures so steadfastly tend to strife that to deprive them of conflict and violence is to do them violence and to sink them in conflict with themselves. They would, in the afterlife, continue rankling. If the choice was theirs, they would much rather bite, and stab, and cudgel than hover in intemporal glory. Like Orlando, they would continue to fight as dead bodies. Boiardo, fifteenth-century Italian poet, tells us that his hero did not really mind being dead:

Così colui del colpo non accorto
Andava combattendo e era morto
(Orlando innamorato, bk. 2, canto 24)

In other words, struck by a hatchet blow, Orlando has just been cut in half. Nonetheless, the two halves still cling to each other, and therefore Orlando can disregard the slight inconvenience of death and continue to thrust and parry blows in the middle of the fray.

But even these fiends die. Once, in Canada, I performed an autopsy on one of them. He was a half-caste American Indian, a member of I know not what tribe. Two students, a morgue attendant, and I strenuously labored for a long time before we succeeded in dragging his body to the autopsy table. Once positioned, his grizzly-bear frame overflowed the sides of the table, and his arms hung like two felled oaks, thicker than the thighs of an average person. This brawny giant had been a lumberjack in the eastern North American uplands, the kind I hitherto believed a purely mythical figure of Canadian folklore. Somewhere in those woods he developed a bull's neck (wider at its base than the diameter of his head at the temples), the most powerful shoulders I ever saw, and such a handgrip as would let him clear a patch of forest with an axe in the time it took two men armed with power saws to do the job. To herculean strength he joined an irksome disposition. A comrade lumberjack, upset at losing a bet, accused him of illegally winning an arm-wrestling match against two simultaneous opponents. In the heat of the discussion he dared to call him a cheat, whereupon he was swiftly pawed on the face and had his nose crushed into comminuted bits. This experience forever changed his physiognomy, enhanced his caution, but did not abate his rancor. After he recovered, he went to his cabin, fetched the ancient shotgun with which he used to stalk his quarry, approached our giant stealthily, and sprayed him point-blank with a burst of pellets. New Orlando, the presumptive victim, hardly blinked; he seemed to care as much for this trivial annoyance as he would have for insistent gnats flying about him. Though bleeding from multiple perforations, he still found the strength to soberly admonish his attacker on the evils of vindictiveness; in what way, I do not know, but in terms so efficacious that the would-be assassin never recovered from his lesson, and our man, who did not die this time, was awarded several years rest in confinement as the prize for his unexampled preaching.

The clinical history was skimpy of nonmedical facts, but it informed us that after his prison term the brawny giant no longer pleased himself in his native land. He roamed far and wide and eventually arrived in the port of Halifax, where he helped in loading and unloading ships. In less time than it takes to tell larboard from starboard, he fell in love with the seafaring life. Because he could single-handedly coil ropes and scrub decks for an entire crew, a boatswain soon was found to sign him up in a merchant ship. Thenceforth, the giant's restlessness had the whole world for its theater. He raged in tavern brawls from Antofagasta to Macao. He crushed Asiatic crania, loosened American teeth, and fractured African ribs. He tattooed his body with figures of winged serpents, odalisques, flower motifs, and the Canadian maple leaf super-scribed with the name of a woman. When he worked at the halyards his muscles tensed, and an entire fauna and flora became animated on his epidermis; and with the rhythmic pulls of hoisting a load, the odalisques shimmied their hips provocatively. In every brothel of the Orient his ornamented nudity caused a general commotion. In Hong Kong, where he would hire three prostitutes per night, a fight broke out among the three over the symbolic meaning of the skin in-scriptions, for none but the Oriental mind is sensitive to the encoded message of patterned decoration. In Malaysia, throngs of natives never failed to crowd the wharves when his ship touched port; with gasping fascination they would watch the giant pulling on the hawser and securing his vessel unassisted. It is no small irony that this titan in the end succumbed to a tiny worm, scarcely three millimeters long. The tapeworm echinococcus found its way into his tissues, and its larvae formed cysts in his liver and in his brain. I may be excused for dispensing with the details of his echinococcosis, which in itself was not unique, and which I have largely forgotten. What I do remember is the massive, gigantic frame, the maple leaf superscribed with the name of one Letitia, and the huge scar left by the gash he once received in Cape Horn at the hands of those who naively thought they might subdue him by force; I hereby declare that no human blow could have broken that skull, which we entered only after long and arduous work with a motor-powered saw. And I also remember, as the anatomical dissection proceeded, the repeated encounter with shotgun pellets imbedded in his tissues; they were present in chest muscles, pleura, lung, pericardium, and even in the substance of the heart, everywhere surrounded by a fibrous tissue capsule, with which the body had successfully segregated these foreign objects from the delicate environment of the organism. As each new pellet was found under the scalpel, we exclaimed: "Here is another one!" dropping the find into a stainless-steel basin, where each pellet fell with a metallic tinkling, until the basin overflowed and we ceased counting. The man had roamed and sailored and brawled and wenched for twenty years, carrying inside nearly a pound of lead. He could have been used for an anchor. For most of his adult life his entire being, save for his moral course, had traveled well ballasted.

By coincidence, at about this time I read the disputes of the early fathers of the Church concerning the problem of bodily identity on the Day of Resurrection. The main contention was that the identity of the body should be preserved on Judgment Day, because it could not be that souls that sinned in one body would be punished in another, nor did it seem fair that a martyr would suffer in one body and be rewarded in another. Resurrection, the actual process of bodily reconstitution, did not present any logical difficulties. As Saint Jerome put it, just as the seeds contain the trunk, boughs, fruit, and leaves, so do the dead contain the seed-plot of the body, which will be instinct with life on the final day. The problem was, Which body would be restored? Would it be our selfsame body? Would its identity be preserved in an absolute fashion? I could thus assume that my Indian, on the authority of Saint Jerome, was going to appear before the heavenly tribunal with his original 3.5-cm-thick calvarium, his very own oxen musculature, and even, perhaps, his epidermal graphics intact. For when Scripture announces that the hour is to come in which the dead "shall hear the voice of the Son of God and shall come forth" (John 5:25), Jerome understands this to mean they shall hear with their own ears, shall come forth on their own feet to comply with the express commandment. Resurrection cannot mean, says the anchorite in his letter to Pammachius, that one thing is destroyed and another raised up. Saint Jerome felt for the body, for *this* body, an attachment that anatomists and pathologists easily understand. However, his viewpoint was not universally accepted among theologians. Origen held precisely the opposite view. He maintained that to press for absolute corporeal identity is heresy. To regain our same parts implies to recover them complete with their respective wants. Irately he asks his opponent: "Do you demand that there should be flesh, bones, blood, limbs, so that you may have the barber to cut your hair, that your nose may run, your nails must be trimmed, your lower parts may gender filth and minister to lust?"

Alas, I never thought of that. According to Origen, we

can never be the same again—even on Judgment Day. We cannot keep our generational organs, or any other organs for that matter, separate from their physiology and their needs. Origen, woefully ignored by medical historians, here makes the first, strongest, and most dramatic case for structure-function correlation. The organ cannot be without its function. Hence, preservation of absolute bodily identity on Judgment Day would be to smuggle a corruptible body into heaven. But this is impossible. Hence, the body shall be "different": not our very own, but one unperceived and wholly ethereal. Hence, my Indian, as I knew him, cannot enter the heavenly kingdom, even assuming he had deserved it. Certainly not with the name of Letitia conspicuously displayed on his chest.

But what if Jerome was in the right? Uncompromising corporealist that he was, he never gave up the belief that our own limbs will sustain us before the heavenly tribunal. We shall have our own eyes and our own ears and our own all-the-rest, he insisted. Yes, in point of fact there shall be sex organs, so "John will be John and Mary will be Mary." But, not to worry: there can be no fear of promiscuity, for we shall be granted the blessedness of angels without ceasing to be human. The author of the Vulgate rhetorically asks: "Who ever crowned a stone for continuing a virgin? Who can have any glory from a life of chastity if we had no sex which would make unchastity possible?" Thus, in Jerome's heaven sex exists as an unrealized potential. In which case, it goes without saying, heaven is out for my seafaring friend.

Since the day we autopsied that giant, many a quarrelsome individual has come under our scalpel. Fierce legions: people of so stubborn a combativeness that in many cases they perished on its account. Out they went, kicking, panting, and raging. It cannot be said that they were laid to rest. Nor can it be assumed that their current abode should be called

OUACHITA TECHNICAL COLLEGE

"final resting place." If it is true, as some believe, that the passage from life to death brings out the truest part of our self, a race of men will continue to do battle in the nether world. Legend and history attest to this, as in the following examples.

Among the Norsemen, whose bellicosity was proverbial, everlasting peace was all but desirable. In the fifth book of *Historia danica*, Saxo Grammaticus recounts the story of two Norse chieftains, Assueit and Asmund, led by friendship to agree that if one should be slain in battle, the other would consent to be buried with his friend. Assueit was killed, whereupon Asmund was entombed with him. A century passed, and then a band of Swedish warriors appeared in the valley. Having heard the story, they decided to open the sepulcher. The idea was to appropriate for themselves the swords, shields, helmets, and other objects with which Norse chiefs were interred in those days. No sooner had they laid aside the big stones and heaped earth that guarded the entrance of the tomb than the air was filled with, instead of the expected sepulchral silence, the clangor of clashing shields and swords, and horrid cries of battle. Where others might have fled in terror, the Norse warriors stood their ground, ready to brave the dead. One of their number was lowered into the tomb at the end of a rope to investigate. And when the signal was given to pull the rope, who should appear in the light of day but the great Asmund, who told in improvised verses the saga of his century-long battle with his quondam friend and immediately thereafter fell dead in front of the travelers. Asmund and Assueit had made a convenant of friendship. But to be reduced to the tomb's inactivity, and to find it intolerable, was all one. Notwithstanding the fact that he was dead, Assueit took up arms against his friend. The combat lasted for one hundred years, at the end of which time Asmund succeeded in reducing his feisty companion to the stillness befitting a corpse by driving a pointed stick into his chest. Then, as if to ensure that Assueit's burial-proof mischief should not recur, his corpse was burned and the ashes scattered. The lot that fell to Asmund was to occupy, alone, the burial site originally built for two.

It must be said in fairness that the belligerence of dead Norsemen was not always wholly unrestrained. In the *Erybiggia Saga* there is a tale of specters who haunted a castle in Iceland. By degrees they took possession of the entire mansion. The frightened owners soon found themselves displaced to the areas of the castle remotest from the fireplace. In Iceland, as one can easily imagine, this uncivil behavior on the part of ghosts was simply criminal. The owners complained to an assembled jury. There was a trial at which the ghosts were present, and judgment went against them. Uttering their choicest dolorous howls, dragging their most sonorous chains, the ghosts vanished never to be seen or heard from again. Sir Walter Scott commented on this strange narrative and remarked that only in the northern European countries, so proud of their jury system, does one find examples of ghosts who enter into suits of eviction and, having lost them, obey the law that forces them to abandon the places they came to haunt!

It may yet be objected that these and other stories do nothing to demonstrate the persistence of individual combativeness in the afterlife. For there are some who place no reliance on legends and folk stories and credit only that set of legends-with-chronology that goes by the name of official history. Photographs, documents, and other dated illusions are what they need. So be it. This naive form of disbelief is easiest to counter, for the world is brimful of the sort of proof that is demanded. As an example, the following story goes a long way to convert the recalcitrant. It is not a legendary account from misty Norwegian marshes nor one of which time has smudged the contours and shaded the outlines. It occurred in sunny Mexico, and people may still be living who could vouch for its truthfulness. It comes from the elegantly sober pen of Martin Luis Guzmán, chronicler of the Mexican Revolution and personal witness to some of its major cataclysms.[1]

William Benton was an Englishman settled in Mexico, the possessor of substantial landholdings when the Revolution exploded. General Villa's troops appeared at his hacienda. The general himself notified him that his property was confiscated by the nation and that he was to be duly compensated for his loss. Benton answered arrogantly and, to his misfortune, attempted to resist. He was disarmed and manacled. General Villa asked his friends what to do. All fell silent except his notorious henchman, Rodolfo Fierro, who was quite direct: The Englishman supported the enemies of the Revolution; he tried to kill Villa. He should be made to pay for his crimes. Should this rich man, on account of being a foreigner, be left unpunished? This persuaded Villa. He ordered that the prisoner be taken away and executed.

The prisoner and a posse of soldiers came down from a train. Straightaway the soldiers started digging. Benton was heard to say: "Listen, *amigos*, dig deeper, or the coyotes will soon dig me out." A sentence that demonstrates, says Villa in his memoirs, that the said Englishman was *un hombre de mucha ley* (a man of great courage). While Benton watched the digging, Fierro came behind him and shot him through the skull.

Only two days had passed when Villa was confronted for the first time by the power of mass media. The international press, fanned by the anti-Revolution faction, accused him of murder. The American consul obtained an interview and apprised the general, in no uncertain terms, of the serious consequences of that death. In candor, Villa told him that the Englishman had been executed.

And who sentenced him to death?

"The Revolutionary Army, *señor*, which is the expression of the people. But it was no murder, for he agreed that what we did was right. He told me that I was going to see that Englishmen, too, know how to die. He did not die in discord with me. He even trusted me to distribute the proceeds of his estate among his relatives, which I have already done."

But what about the corpse?

"It is buried."

Can we recover it?

"Yes, *señor*. After some time."

Is the grave well marked, that it should not get lost?

"My graves never get lost, *señor*."

Days later, a special envoy of the United States government appeared before Villa demanding an official transcript of the trial of William Benton.

"And why should you demand papers, when my word is as good as gold?"

The foreign agent, Mr. George C. Carothers, explained to General Villa that he, or his government, had always trusted Villa's word. However, the great powers were desirous of extinguishing the flame of the Revolution. Unless their demand was satisfied, there was danger of foreign intervention, which would be to the grave detriment of the rebels' cause. Villa then summoned the lawyers that accompanied the famed Northern Division.

"See to it that an official transcript is produced, wherein the details of the execution of Benton by the revolutionary forces appear properly recorded."

In the midst of his military campaigns, Villa received a surprising telephone call. An international commission had been formed demanding the exhumation of Benton's remains. The exhumed body was to be surrendered to his widow.

"Why should we do that? They cannot force us. The widow is a Mexican national."

Not so. Having married a Briton, she had been extended the same protection Imperial Britain grants all born under its flag. It was therefore explained to the general that European interests colluded to exert great pressure upon the government of the United States. President Wilson himself, together with his secretary of state, had specifically directed the newly appointed commission to carry out the business with the greatest possible expediency.

To compound his consternation, Villa now learned that Benton was never placed in front of a firing squad.

"*Amiguitos*, here is what you will do: You are to unearth the body of Benton from where you placed it. You are to bury it in the Regla Cemetery of the City of Chihuahua. The International Commission will disinter it from there, and they must see plain evidence that Benton was executed by a firing squad."

William Benton, wherever you might be today, receive our sincere homage! Boiardo's stanzas could not extoll your prowess, for they sang of a hero who continued to fight out of forgetfulness, whereas you held armies in check knowing full well that you were dead. Let your name survive—and let it be for the admiration of posterity—as a reminder of the only corpse so mettlesome that it could not be subdued simply by murder and burial but had to be unearthed, executed twice, and twice buried!

The International Commission never got Benton's spoils. Alarmed at the consequences of the rising international scandal, President Carranza firmly barred Villa from further participation in this matter. In place of the unsophisticated general, the chief command appointed slick lawyers from Mexico City and diplomats wise in the ways of international dispute, who refused to negotiate with England on the grounds that it had broken diplomatic relationships with Mexico, and with the United States on the grounds that the incident concerned England only. The story of the cadaver sentenced to death by posthumous shooting was not released until Villa's memoirs were published.

OF SOME BODILY
APPENDAGES

T HERE is an unequal apportionment of historical prestige
to the various parts of the anatomy. In all times, at all
places, segments of our body were ennobled even as others
were vilified. Almost without exception the heart was made
the residence of sentiment, exalted as the motor that impels
the cogs and wheels of a wondrous creation. The liver, which
modern physiology commits to the role of semi-industrial, if
amazingly sophisticated, warehouse and chemical processor,
has been taken for the seat of combativeness, of melancholy,
of love, and even as the mooring that fastens the soul to the
perishable body. Its latin name (Sp.: *hígado*, It.: *fegato*), still
recognizable in the word *hepatic*, derives from vulgar Latin
ficatum (because geese used to be overfed with a diet of figs
to render their livers fatty). The Italian writer Ceronetti thus
observes that behind the most common anatomical works
there is often an inglorious record of man's inhumanity.[1]

All that is noble and excellent and all that is worst in
human commerce has been thought to derive from the brain,
a sort of gland that secretes lofty ideas and superior morals
when healthy and oozes destructive plans when diseased. And
even those anatomical formations whose ledger might include
a sum total of folly and devastation possibly exceeding their

survival value, like the genital organs, have been romanticized by folklore, deified by pagan religions, and abhorred by puritans. Hippocrates taught that the uterus was mobile, its restless wanderings charting the course of feminine pathos; and long after the absurdity of a traveling womb was questioned, the learned continued to believe that its emanations were the cause of hysteria.

Other organs were perhaps deemed too humble to be surrounded by mystery and superstition or crowned by the tales of folklore. Our ancestors seemed to have been concerned but little with the thyroid gland or the lymph nodes, whose magic is entirely contemporary. But of those anatomical parts that the nonphysiologist can readily see, the lore is inexhaustible.

The nose, for example, symbolized character, as the eyes were supposed to show forth its inner movements: short and upturned in the prim; angular and strong in the temerarious; regular in the just; sharp and daggerlike in the devious. To our day, nose is destiny; and to be born with a nose that disclaims its owner is a very real tragedy, a kind of biological-metaphysical tug-of-war. Each of us is, as in the Spanish verse *"hombre a una nariz pegado,"* a mere appendix to the dominant entity of the self: the nose, the true repository of individual identity. This is why a man of genius, if he happens to have anything other than an average nasal appendage, will not fail to feel its keen domination. Gogol is said to have been proud of being capable of touching the tip of his nose with his lower lip, a contortionist's feat that he achieved thanks as much to his vaunted muscular elasticity as to the fact that his nose, judging from his portraits, terminated in a downward bird's bill-like promontory. To this accident of birth (the obscure ways of Providence are still called "accidents") we owe the short story "The Nose," in which Kovalyov discovers one day that this nose has left him. In a sequence that anticipates surrealism, Gogol alternatively surprises us, saddens us, and amuses us, narrating the vicissitudes of a bold nose that decides to pursue its own life, climbs into a carriage to seek its fortune in the world, and leaves behind its dejected and confused former owner, who looks in consternation at his new flat, barren, level, noseless face reflected in the mirror.

Vladimir Nabokov has written pages of scholarly disquisition on what he called Gogol's "olfactivism."[2] He informs us that an obsession with the nose is rightfully a Russian prerogative, for the nose, long before Gogol's short story, had conquered the Russian mind. Thus we are told that more than other peoples, Russians refer to the nose in proverbs, sayings, and humor: if dejected, they hang it down; if elated, they lift it up; if forgetful, they notch it to help memory, as we tie strings around our fingers; if visited by good news, their nose will itch; if by amorous dalliance, a nasal pimple will show it. I was delighted by the Russian definition of a big nose as one that can bridge the Volga, for it would be difficult to think of a more vigorous image of power and span than this one, built to oppose the might of nature. But I am less ready to concede that Russians have been any more percipient of the power and magic of the nose than other peoples. At least in the West (I am reminded that the Chinese, comparatively less endowed with nasal protuberance, use the expression *dà-bidz*, "big nosed," as a pejorative reference to Westerners) all abide by the nasal ethos. And the strife between nose and spirit has spawned a rich literature that may be called epic, given its sweep and intensity.

Cyrano de Bergerac, the Homer of olfactivism, lends voice to the conflict of the soul that would like to soar in its aspiration of love and spirituality but is instead betrayed by a deformed nose that weights it down to triviality and denial. In desperation, he creates a mythical extraterrestrial race of long-nosed men in whom nasal length is directly proportional to virtue. A visitor to their planet asks the time and is answered with a grimace that uncovers the teeth: the nose is used as a gnomon that projects its shadow on the dental sundial. The nose thus acquires the utility of a practical device in addition to its symbolic utility as the banner of probity. And when the visitor wishes to know how nasal hypertrophy became the universal feature of all citizens of the model republic, it is explained to him that every newborn child is taken to the temple by the midwife, where a committee of experts compares the length of the infant's nose with a unit of measure held by the syndic. If the nose falls short of this standard, the infant is adjudicated pug-nosed and castrated forthwith. And if the visitor should feel inclined to regard this measure as barbarous and paradoxical in a country that looks upon virginity as a crime, the following explanation is offered: thirty centuries of observation have led to the conclusion that a prominent nose is the unfailing "marker" of spirituality, courtesy, generosity, and prudence in its possessor, whereas a small nose is equally specific for the vices that stand in opposition to these qualities. Hence, it is in the public interest to make eunuchs out of these pug-nosed individuals rather than take the risk of possible deterioration of the race.[3]

An idle writer who wished to compile a purely literary anthology of a single anatomical organ would find the task infinite. Of the less well-known organs he would find a vast tradition of fear and awe; of external anatomical regions, an endless projection of people's ignorance, fancies, and empirical observations bordering on science. Even insensitive, dispensable appendages, inert formations of the living self, like nails or hair would be found ensconced in a massive weave of legend: the former traveling as relics of saints or ensheathed in richly inlaid cases and flaunted as symbols of mandarin supremacy; the latter braided into long tresses as ropes for suitors to climb towers with. But is this true for every part of the human anatomy? What about, say, the sacrococcygeal region, i.e., the lowest back, backside, rear end, behind, rump, derriere? Could it be that an area of the human body has been reserved strictly for ridicule or off-color vulgarity? No rhapsodies here; no lyricism. Our diligent anthologist would have to wade through enormous bogs of softcover mud, enormous expanses of filth that would take him from the most sordid lupanar to the palatial mansion of the archbishop of Lyon, where Sade, the *philosophe scélérat* had Mme Lacroix display her rotund behind to His Eminence in a perversely baroque curtsy.

It is not often that the imagination of writers fails to recognize the hieratic mystery of a human bodily part. But in the case of the sacrococcyx, literary flights utterly missed their target: the backside has been the material substratum of ridicule to comedians or the recourse of cheap tantalizing to pornographers. It is, to the biologist, much more than that. This remote province of the organism, this target of bastinades and kicks in every buffoon that ever trod the stage is actually a crossroads of cellular life, a cosmopolis of the human economy, a kaleidoscopic center of growth and potential energy. This potential is revealed only in disease, but when disease manifests, what a nightmarish, fantastic pathology! By comparison the brain or the heart appear ridiculously provincial. A tumor developing in the questionably "noble" organs will almost always be composed of tissues indigenous to their structure. But a tumor of the sacrococcygeal region, at least in children, usually results in a chaotic mass of tissues of every description. As if the rearend were the great planifier and mastermind of the body—which it may be, our cephalocentric prejudice notwithstanding—the resulting tumor mass (teratoma) displays the formation of brain, bowel, teeth, hair, endocrine glands, and all tissues that under normal circumstances are sparingly and fastidiously bred, but this time chaotically and luxuriantly bursting forth. The terms that medical men have used in connection with the caudal end of the developing body, such as "organizer" or "totipotential," ring of the reverence and awe that literary men have systematically denied to this maligned bit of our own selves.[4]

Still another form of deviancy, less exuberant than a teratoma, is the formation of a caudal appendix. This pathology, though innocuous and much less complex than a teratoma, is equally spectacular and somehow more disturbing. For what are we to think of a tailed man? Or, rather, what are we to think of ourselves and our cherished notion of evolutionary superiority, seeing that one of us can be born tailed? In more pious times, an explanation was not difficult to find. In England it was believed that the men of Kent were born tailed in payment for the inhabitants of the village of Strood having insulted the disgraced Thomas Becket, carrying their show of disrespect to the point of cutting the tail of the prelate's horse. Says Andrew Marvell in "The Loyal Scot":

> *There's no - Deliver us from a bishop's wrath.*
> *Never shall Calvin pardon'd be for sales,*
> *Never, for Burnet's sake, the Lauerdales;*
> *For Becket's sake, Kent always shall have tails.*

John Bayle, bishop of Ossory under Edward VI, admitted a second version: "For castynge of fyshe tayles at thys Augustine, Dorsettshyre men had tayles ever after." Somehow, a high sense of fair play may have led Englishmen to expect that there should be tailed men amongst them after the mentioned infamy. Scarcely sixty or seventy years ago, children of that country still believed that all Cornishmen were born with tails, never questioning how the curse of Kent passed into the West country. English nannies may have perpetuated the medieval belief, in which, as John Bayle put it, "They have diffamed the English posterity with tails. That an Englishman now cannot travayle in another land by way of marchandayse or any other occupying, but it is most contumeliously thrown in his tethe that all Englishmen have tails."

Baring-Gould carefully scrutinized the accumulated descriptions of tailed human beings, from the quaint to the grotesque, only to conclude in ponderous, turn-of-the-century style, that tails were a biologic impossibility in human beings, "for the spine terminates in the os sacrum, a large and expanded bone of peculiar character, entirely precluding all possibility of production to the spine as in caudate animals." He could have abbreviated with the sober admonition of Doctor Johnson: "Of a standing fact, sir, there ought to be no controversy; if there are men with tails, catch a *homo caudatus*." Today we know that the catches have been numerous. Trapped by photography, the strange specimens are exhibited in plenty of case reports. One of these was entitled "Baby with a Tail"; the subtitle, carefully following the instructions to authors anent space limitations and descriptive pith, read: "And he could wag it, too!" For the benefit of the scientifically inclined, there is a recent update on *homo caudatus*. This was the only catch of the Boston Children's Hospital Medical Center between 1936 and 1982, noted in an article published in the prestigious *New England Journal of Medicine*. A healthy baby was born with a tail that measured 5.5 cm in length by 0.7 cm in diameter at its base, tapering toward the tip, and emerged 1.5 cm to the right of the midline adjacent to the sacrum; histological examination showed it to be composed of skin tissues only, having neither cartilage nor bone. To the casual observer it looked like a large and well-formed tail. But it was boneless and off-center. Thus, in the best scientific tradition it was pronounced a tail and not a tail. The scholarly discussion in the report is admirable in its breadth, summoning arguments from embryology, biochemistry, genetics, and comparative anatomy. In the course of the discussion it is mentioned that, from the standpoint of molecular biology, we are closer to our tailed animal brethren than we would like to think. Thus, there is an astounding similarity between human and chimpanzee DNA, as there is between the chimpanzee's genome and that of other primates, including tailed monkeys. If we are phenotypically different, it seems, we owe it to regulatory genes rather than structural genes. In the best scientific tradition, it is concluded that the appearance of a tail in a human baby should be interpreted as a regression and not a regression.[5]

It seems rather surprising that this anatomical region, used in literary circles mainly for laughs or leers, is defined by biology as the palaestra for the mighty clash between creationists and evolutionists.

MYASIS

T HE PATIENT was a young man who had known, at one time, the shelter and comfort of a middle-class North American home. The tide of life severed him thence. How and why he became a chronic derelict of society was thought to be irrelevant to his hospitalization. For some time he had been sleeping under bridges or on rooftops. Long remiss in the care of his own person, he ate rarely, either from trashcans or petty thefts at markets. With indifference more than covertly akin to suicide, he threw himself into alcoholic binges, one of which left him comatose in the middle of the street. Solicitous public officials, more concerned with the antiesthetic effects of an unkempt body lying athwart the city traffic than with that body's ultimate fate, material or spiritual, picked him up and left him at the emergency room of a county hospital.

His bodily surface showed signs of scabies, malnutrition, local skin pigmentation suggestive of pellagra, and infection. All findings were recorded with the usual unflinching professionalism; one, however, caused even the least squeamish to recoil: tiny whitish ovoid bodies, writhing with spontaneous sinuous motions, emerged from sinus tracts that opened to the inflamed skin surface of the patient's legs. A biopsy proved that the parasite in question was none other than the ubiquitous fly; the common, familiar, domestic fly. Larval forms of *Musca domestica.*

Much gesturing, rue, and lamentation flowed, on that occasion, from the hospital staff. One heard, on that day, that to become a vehicle for such filthy insects was a mark of the ultimate misery; no human abjection greater than this could be imagined. Yet the truth in such statements may be challenged. Parasitism is but one among myriad forms of suffering, a biologic encounter at which, sooner or later, we are all to suffer defeat. That a man should have been so humbled by the fly is apparently uncommon but certainly not degrading. Perchance the encounter was staged between a biologic overlord and its natural vassal. But who is lord and who is vassal? This assignment of roles does not conform to our wishes.

For all the gesturing and queasiness that accompanied the diagnostic proceedings, the common fly is by no means contemptible. She may be the smallest of winged creatures, but as Lucian reminds us, not the humblest, for she takes precedence even of kings in eating and swaggers about on their tables and tastes all they are to eat . . . after she is satisfied. It was not in vain that the Greeks explained her origin, if not on a par with the gods, at least brought forth by divine mediation. Μυιαν (the fly) was originally a beautiful girl, though one garrulous and prattling in the extreme. Her love for Endymion only increased her garrulousness and made her outgoing beyond propriety. She kept paying him inopportune visits and generally making herself a nuisance. Instead of capturing the attention of Endymion, she merely succeeded in making Selene jealous. Selene, without further ado, turned her into the fly we know. Which is why, Lucian tells us, "in remembrance of Endymion she begrudges all sleepers their repose, especially those of tender years." With this background, however, we know that her biting and provocation are not cruel harassment, but the tokens of love and friendship.

As time passed, the vicissitudes of the fly continued. She was caught in the cross fire when Saint Augustine undertook his mettlesome defense of the City of God; all the pagan deities were then locked out of the citadel and turned into pathetic beggars. Excessive want, it is well known, brings out the worst in us. Those who once were carefree Olympians, carousing and playing pranks immune to human judgment, became maleficent demons reduced to pounding on the doors of the citadel, forever shut before them. Inside the citadel, where Μυιαν chanced to find herself, all who could have Olympian-pagan connections became suspect. It was Luther who accused her of being part of the fifth column. Where Lucian had heard a melodious droning, "sweeter than the music of cymbals and flutes," Luther perceived the ominous buzzing of the Evil One; and her persistent attacks, which Lucian saw as caused by her undying love for Endymion, Luther interpreted as the stubborn harassment of the Devil. To Luther there could be no question that the Devil had slipped into his house in the guise of a fly with the specific mission of distracting him, as Bertrand Russell observes, "from writing good books." Our own age is less preoccupied with the question of the divine or infernal nature of the fly. But surely it is one or the other.

Consider her eyes: Whereas we see the world through the simple translucency of smoothly curved corneas, the compound eyes of a fly, with thousands of hexagonal facets, or ommatidial units, collect light rays inciding upon them from infinite angles and catch we know not what indescribable iridescences. The perfection of our own sense organs is a wonder, but each time we compare these faculties with the exquisite organization of the special senses of individuals of humbler species, we are invariably struck more by the limitations than the strengths of our faculties. The rate of flicker at which light appears continuous will still be lower in man (45–53 per second) than in some insects (250 per second or more); and the sensitivity to range in wavelength will also be lower, so that flies can see where man is blind—in the ultraviolet part of the spectrum. Should we brag about our capacity to integrate stereoscopic images in our much-vaunted brain cortex, the fly can retort that she, or members of her family, can read polarized light. And she can project, on her minuscule brain, a fantastic mosaic of thousands of images gathered by her compound eyes, integrating a vision of the world that we can hardly imagine. Only the boldest among us have dared to attempt a reconstruction of this vision, by technics that are generally dangerous. Like Huxley, some have strived to enlarge the Doors of Perception with the hammer-blows of mescaline and by chiseling away with hallucinogens; but all this chipping and hammering away can easily make the mind fly off in pieces, and it is common to observe that the pillars of sanity cave in much before ommatidial vision is attained by those who start off with a regular set of corneas.

The highest services commonly acknowledged in our specialized senses are two. First, reflective people say, no knowledge would be possible without them, for they are irreplaceable devices with which we grasp the external world; and the most simple, as well as the most complicated, explanation of the universe, must always start from an irreducible set of perceptions conveyed by the senses. Second, practical-minded people tell us that the most valuable service rendered by the specialized senses is that of ensuring our survival. In other words, before sitting down to construct a philosophical system, our capacity to see, hear, smell, and touch will direct us to sit *by* the fireplace, not *on* it. This much we have to grant to the fly: that on both counts her senses compare favorably with ours, but on the latter she is much superior to us. For if the noblest function of the senses were to furnish building blocks for our philosophical constructs, there is no reason why a cornerstone with low threshold to flickering light should be better than one of higher discrimination in this regard. Our judgment should be confined, needless to say, to the building blocks and not to the completed edifice, for we know that it is the nature of one philosophical system to be impermanent, and that one must be toppled by another in endless series, and that none is definite. But if the highest function of the senses is what pragmatic people suggest, namely, to ensure survival, then the matter is settled: the fly comes out the uncontested winner. She was there in prehistoric times, long before man, as attested by fossils that trace everything from narrow waist to wing venation, and she will be there long after man ceases to be. Indeed, those who picture Armageddon as a heap of corpses left in the wake of nuclear war, famine, and disease paint an incomplete semblance. If they look closer, they will find the heap of carrion teeming with maggots—the future flies.

Consider *Sarcophaga*, the flesh fly, hovering above the decomposing corpses. Now and then she alights on the dank recesses of the rotting body and deposits myriads of larvae expelled from her generational organs into the slimy, fetid soup that builds up in the crevices of the cadaver. Consider this brood, each one provided with a floating device, a kind of life buoy that will enable it to float on carrion soup, while the "breathing cups" placed at its caudal extremity and shaped like a diadem keep opening and closing to enable respiration. Fabre, the entomologist, compared the floating coronet of the grub to a tiny flower: its denticulations he compared to petals, and the breathing holes at the bottom, to stamens. In the writhing of maggots on decomposing meat he thought he saw the beauty of an unbroken shoal of sea anemones! The fly taught Fabre and his readers, if nothing more, that most sobering of lessons about beauty and the eye of the beholder. An insistent question posed by the fly is also a very old one. It is the question of guessing the purpose of so peculiar a creature's existence. It is almost a necessity to suppose that so much contrivance in living beings is a work of design, and hard to accept that it might be the work of chance. Strictly speaking, one does not need the fly to come to grips with the question of purpose in the Creation. In fact, we have behind us a long history of conceit that has made it unnecessary for us to look elsewhere than ourselves to be struck with wonder at the stupendous ingeniousness of our own design and thence to conclude that such an elaborate machinery "must" have issued from a conscientious and loving creator. Xenophon, in his *Memorabilia* (bk. 1, ch. 4, sec. 6) reminisces of a Socratic tirade, not without comic details: It is a wonder that our delicate eyes should be provided with a canopy of eyelashes to filter harmful sunrays; that they should be surmounted by a copse of eyebrows to catch the drops of sweat that might cause irritation. It is a wonder that we should have nostrils in close proximity to the eyes, to catch the odor of what we see. It is amazing that our ears can catch all sounds without being choked by them. It seems prodigious that the mouth should be so close to the other sense organs, so as to admit what through our other senses we desire . . . "but since what goes out is unpleasant, the ducts through which it passes are turned away and removed as far as possible from the organs of sense. With such signs of forethought in these arrangements, can you doubt whether they are the works of chance or of design?" No, of course not, had to answer Aristodemus the dwarf to this rhetorical question.

Our senses, regarded in this light, look like the handiwork of a wise and loving creator. But what about the fly's? She gloats upon the excrementitious residues that we detest. She thrives on pus, on decomposed blood, on organic fluid oozing from wounds and sores. Among close to eighty-five thousand species of two-winged insects that we may call *flies*, there are some who colonize the anal orifice of cattle—and would fain choose ours for habitat were it not that we keep it, as Quevedo used to say, "enshrouded and buried in life"; and there are some that avidly lap tears and nasal secretions, and swarm about the faces of neglected babies and indigent adult human beings; and many that have a stylet for proboscis, the better to indulge in blood sucking; and many more who carry bacteria and viruses deadly to us. Epidemiologists have estimated that one-quarter of all the mortality in the world is fly related.

Thus the fly reminds us, lest we are too prompt to conclude that the entire creation is to be taken as a gift for our unalloyed enjoyment, that together with a most admirable contrivance in our design, provisions were made for our decay and suffering. Not the least of these is an army of eighty-five thousand battalions of Diptera that systematically fells roughly 25 percent of our number every generation. The fly compels us more insistently than the lark or the tree, because she is truly ubiquitous, to ponder the old, old question of chance versus design in things and living beings as we encounter them in the world. But between an individual case of myasis and the problem of a cosmic purpose underlying the universe, the chasm is too wide and too deep; becoming dizzy, I prefer to let the matter rest here.

THE BODY FROM OUTSIDE

(With Notes on the Outside of the Inside)

CONSIDER the body from outside. This mass of thews and sinews, this conglomerate of skin-covered angles and rotundites, of animated prominences and quivering hollows, invariably affects the observer with a strong impact. Whether a positive or a negative one, it seems to depend entirely on the viewer's temperament.

If the esthetic sense is but slightly developed, the imagination is bound to be captured whole. In the body's formal beauty, in its movement, in its plastic expression, lies a fascination that the artist can easily exalt to the quality of religious worship. Greco-Roman sculptors did not hesitate; they went ahead, untrammeled by any discouring notion, to a celebration of the human body as the luminous starting and ending point of the natural universe. Christian artists, already schooled in the idea that what is naturally decaying is not a proper subject of worship, had to wait for the Renaissance to dust off the pagan sarcophagi, along with their own ill-repressed hedonism. But then the celebration of the human body exploded with a strength all the more spectacular on account of long postponement. In Michelangelo's *Battle of Cascina* we can see that it came back with a vengeance, juxtaposing bodies in every conceivable attitude under the flimsiest pretext; in his *Battle of Centaurs* the celebration, like a three-staged liturgy, explodes, echoes, and reverberates, respectively, in three different planes of stone. And the exuberant fireworks of Venetians, Florentines, and Romans touched off the celebration elsewhere. Prelates who taught the disdain of the flesh were to shudder at the unveiling of triptychs that, square in the middle of their northern churches, illustrated their sermons of renunciation with the symbols of the most plangent paganism: swooning Madonnas that might have been ravished nymphs or ecstatic Ledas; cherubs that might have passed for Cupids. Muscular satyrs, complete with pointed ears, were still posing as the hired hands who raised the cross and lowered the body of our Savior in Antwerp's altarpiece, at the time of Rubens. Such is the expressive power of the body that even the fathers of the Church are said to have appropriated the fallacy that reads the qualities of the soul on the appearance of the temporal body; thus Saint Ambrose stated: *Species corporis simulacrum est mentis* (the kind of body reflects the kind of mind), and Saint Augustine seemed to imply that a deformed and repugnant body could hardly reflect a well-composed spirit: *Incomposito corporis inaequalitatem indicat mentis* (a discomposed body indicates a disarranged mind).

Opposed to the idea of body as glory, there is the idea of body as prison. Plotinus, a pagan, regretted being "encased" in the body by nature. He refused to sit for painters or sculptors, arguing that it was coercion enough to have to carry this image for the duration of mortal life and that it was sheer nonsense to still wish to "produce a longer lasting image of the image, as if it was something worth looking at." Not that he was without respect for living beings; his biographer, Porphyry, tells us that he refused to eat meat, even as medicine, on the grounds that he believed it wrong to eat the flesh of animals. We are also told that, afflicted with an intestinal disease, he staunchly refused to submit to an enema, saying that it was undignifying for an elderly man to undergo this form of treatment. Thus he was both a philosopher of great stature and a sensible person, able at one time to discern the noble aspects of nature and the merits of Aesculapian Medicine.[1]

Plotinus's spiritual ancestors, the Platonists, fully realized the paradox of a perfect mind, or an intemporal soul, "encased" in a mortal body. Their obsessive love of ideas and the function of the intellect made them confer different degrees of excellence on the component parts of the body. The head, of course, they assumed at the outset to be the "divinest part of us and lord over the rest"; the remainder of the body was seen as mere vehicle for the head's easy movement. Platonic cosmogony saw the gods copying the round shape of the universe to fashion the head, which they made the dwelling place of the divine part of the soul. Fearing its pollution, however, by the base part of the soul, they invented the neck as a sort of isthmus that would keep the divine and mortal soul aliquots asunder. But since the mortal part of the soul has itself a nobler and a baser part, the gods partitioned the trunk with the diaphragm, so as to screen off the site of the "upper mortal soul," in charge of restraining appetites and irrational urges, from the "lower mortal soul," a kind of undomesticated beast that must be fed if the race is to subsist, but that must be kept as far as possible from the head, "the seat of counsel."

In the Platonists' system man is, above all, mind. Man's essence is intellect, and intellect is the most noble reflection from a pure universe of archetypal perfection; thus the whole of the anatomy is made subordinate to the intellect and its function. The divine plan of distribution of the flesh, accordingly, is of a kind that best serves the thinking process. It is all right for compact layers of flesh to wrap themselves around arms, thighs, and hips, for these are areas without intelligence. No such arrangement is conceivable around the head, for it would cause "dullness of sensation in the region of the mind." As for the generational organs, predictably dealt with in a way that is at one time belated and nugatory, they are relegated to the lower compartment. They seem to anticipate Sartre's phrasing in *Diable et le bon Dieu*: "The lower half of the body was made by the devil." In *Timaeus* the language used in reference to the coming into being of the male sex organs is, interestingly, descriptive of an independent being: "self-willed, like a creature deaf to reason and determined, because of frenzied appetite, to carry all before it." The pagan gods, notorious as pranksters, could be expected to place at one end of the human anatomy the elevating impulse of the idea and at the other end a capricious being acting of its own accord to disregard it. Hence the Hellenic traditional partition of Eros: a sublime form of Eros resides in the head, and an uncouth "Eros of begetting" tenants the lower reaches of the anatomy. This schizoid tendency, antedating the Christian era, passed on undiluted to succeeding ages. In at least one case it spilled over into an artist's field of vision, with a most peculiar effect. Such is the example of El Greco.

Having learned his art from the Venetians, El Greco painted bodies that naturally experience all the gravitational pull that earthly beings suffer. Living in the rigidly dogmatic society of Catholic Toledo, they are equally subject to an elevating impulse that would drag them toward the firmament, like disembodied souls that left behind their corporeal "sheaths," just as the famed Toledan sword blades, on the slightest provocation, used to leave their leather encasements with a deadly hissing sound. Caught between irresistible terrestrial and heavenly pulls, El Greco's bodies stretch beyond anything credible. As his angels grow in length, it occurs to him that they need huge wings to be supported in flight. Officers of the Inquisition—not well versed in aeronautics, we are to assume—object to the wing size as contrary to prescribed canons and must be persuaded: "functional" wings or none at all! His kneeling worshippers, his standing figures, stretch to a degree that seems objectionable to most of his contemporaries and, in the saying of Maurice Barrès, "repugnant to many [of ours], who expected to be presented with butterflies transmuted in worship, and are instead presented with long larvae in livid colors."[2]

The Cretan artist who so well expressed the ideals of Spain's Golden Century had to contend, in life and posthumously, with accusations of insanity. It seems that, as time went on, the two opposing pulls were felt more keenly, and the deformation of El Greco's bodies became greater and greater. Barrès tells us of the study by a Spanish erudite, Beritens, entitled "Why El Greco Painted the Way He Painted." Much scholarly effort is made therein to demonstrate that the painter suffered from progressive astigmatism. Through the use of glasses that correct this defect, a counterproof is offered: if one looks at his paintings through such lenses, lo and behold! the proportions will suddenly appear normal. Thus, if we are to believe this thesis, a bad case of genius could have been averted by an opportune visit to the ophthalmologist.

Neither artists nor Platonists agree with the mystic's view of the body. The latter tells us that the body's defining qualities are corruptibility and finiteness. On occasion, an artist might depict decay. A German painter of the first part of this century drew a skeleton, half covered by disintegrating carrion, inside a musty and cobwebbed coffin and entitled it "My self-portrait in 1980." Given the leveling uniformity of death, his rendition probably gained in accuracy with the passage of time. But there seems somehow to be little merit in this sort of artistic foresight, and an artistic career was apparently never based exclusively on such sitters. No one particularly likes the sight of senescence, deformity, or death, yet some are crippled, many reach old age, and all, without exception, are going to die. These truths, which we now rank among platitudes, may come, to some, as sudden and frightening discoveries. In the Indian legend, Siddhartha, a young prince, was confined in a palace for the first twenty-nine years of his life, surrounded by luxury and opulence, with nothing to remind him of the corruptibility of the human body. His father relied on the pleasures of this life and placed no credence in the existence of any other. However, on three successive sallies from the palace, the prince encountered a man bent by old age, a leper, and a dead man being transported to his burial. The shocking realization of the frailty of the human condition made the prince forsake his pleasures, don the yellow robe of the ascetics, and live as a hermit. Thus, Siddhartha became Buddha. Saint John the Damascene, impressed by the beauty of this legend, rewrote, circa 750 A.D., the same legend in the Greek language under the title of *Barlaam and Ioasaph*. In this new version, the young prince Ioasaph is first sobered by the spectacle of corruptibility, and then a monk, Barlaam, takes it upon himself to edify the young man in the truths of the Christian gospel. Let us pardon the Damascene for appropriating, long before the days of copyright, all the details of Sanskrit oral tradition. Because this plagiarism reached worldwide diffusion, Borges observed that Buddha did much to promote and divulgate the Christian gospels.[3]

More than twelve centuries after Barlaam and Ioasaph, it remains difficult to actually believe that the body wears and tears—up to an irreversible point. This is one notion that arrives either as an obscure premonition or a sudden revelation, never as "knowledge," and usually too late. Simone de Beauvoir tells this simple and poignant story of her mother's terminal illness. At one time, with an unsuspected cancer already far advanced, the old woman lies in bed, a lean and sunken frame surrounded by fit, trim physicians bent over her with professional attentiveness. The old woman is not ashamed any more; the time for modesty is past. Gazing upon the naked body of her mother, de Beauvoir writes:

> The sight of my mother's nakedness had jarred me. No body existed less for me: none existed more. As a child I had loved it dearly; as an adolescent it filled me with an uneasy repulsion; all this was perfectly in the ordinary course of things and it seemed reasonable to me that her body should retain its dual nature, that it should be both repugnant and holy—a taboo . . . Only this body, suddenly reduced by her capitulation to being a body and nothing more, hardly differed at all from a corpse—a poor defenceless carcass turned and manipulated by professional hands, one in which life seemed to carry on only because of its own stupid momentum . . . For the first time I saw her as a dead body under suspended sentence. *(A Very Easy Death)*

The mystic's view of the body goes one step further. Since the overriding concern before death is union with the deity, all worldly worries must be shunned; of these, the body's demands are the most imperious and insistent, and so they are the most powerful distracting force that turns us away from the only worthwhile goal. Hence the body is a deadweight that hampers our efforts to ascend to a superior form of life. Hence it, too, must be shunned, or opposed, or ignored. To its demands of satisfaction, we are to counter with privation. Thus a barbarous struggle is established: the body demands food, and the mystic replies by fasting; the body asks for gratification, and the mystic gives mortification. Exasperated, the body will raise visions of banquets, hallucinations of orgies, nightmares of fright. Undaunted, the mystic will renew his self-denial. We think of the haggard, soiled, hirsute medieval monks, oblivious of the blind stubbornness of the body, of the obstinacy with which hair grows, or of the insistence with which the tips of fingers and toes keep growing keratinous appendices, eventually incurved and clawlike. We think of Saint Simon, years atop his scaffold, as unmindful of the vermin accumulating in his tattered robe as of the wistful entreaties of his mother, standing underneath his platform; or of Saint Macarius, who lived on a well and constantly carried about him, to humiliate the insolence of a body that would not cease to crave for pleasure, eighty pounds of irons and chains.

All this, which we call excess, stems from the belief that God cannot be "known" but may be directly experienced, and that such experience is only attainable by the systematic annihilation of all possible bodily distractions. For to lodge God in one's soul is not like housing a transient weekend visitor, for whom casual cleaning would do: the Creator will reclaim the entire soul as his rightful estate, and he is to enter it only after a cleansing so thorough that nothing remains. Thus starts the systematic process that the Zen masters called "ceasing of desires," that Father Jean-Joseph Surin equated to a "holy indifference," and that Aldous Huxley masterfully interpreted for the twentieth-century mentality: a disciplined uprooting of everything, whether in the body or the mind, that might interfere with divine contemplation. Appetites, desires, intellectual curiosity, likes or dislikes, all is to be deleted to make room for the Gift of Grace. This awesome task has inspired admiration or uneasy loathing, never indifference. The former gave birth to panegyrics that underscore our superior nature; the latter to satires that map the absurd proximity of the jurisdictions of the ridiculous and the sublime. With perhaps unsurpassed savagery, the sanguinary pen of Balzac has left us a crassly irreverent sketch of one of the many human beings who misjudged her strength and, aspiring to the ethereal, ended up in buffoonery. In "The Merry Tattle of the Nuns of Poissy," Sister Petronille offers, on the advice of her confessor, every mortification to God. Her constant fasts have rendered her body emaciated and its excreta overly concentrated, "of the hard consistency of deer droppings." One afternoon, after several months, she must relieve the animal body of its excess. Her weakness and the hardness of the stools put her through the most harrowing of "sphincterian terrors." In the midst of her torture, thinking of the merits of this new sacrifice, she exclaims: "Oh God, I offer it to thee!" at the same time the hardened bolus quits her holy person and falls, with the sound of a bouncing rock of flint, into the latrine.

That different observers should hold such different views of the body leads me to believe in Paul Valéry's proposal that there are, in effect, at least four different bodies in each of us. The first one is that which requires an inordinate apportionment for mechanical activity. It is the body that catches the attention of the artist: 20 percent of its external surface taken up by the arms, close to 40 percent by the legs—as if walking, running, leaping, pushing, and hauling were activities deserving of the most onerous evolutionary tribute. The implicit goal of its design is action, a pattern that repeats itself in all the "higher" animal forms, in which wings, tails, fins and forelegs, organs of prehension, propulsion, swimming, or flight take the largest share of the anatomy. The Greeks reflected about this peculiarity: 90 percent of the body adapted for interaction with the environment and 10 percent for judgment and discrimination of its most appropriate kind. Marañón, the Spanish essayist and physician, noted the seeming collaterality of the male's sexual design. It seemed to him as if the pattern had been completed and the Creator, suddenly struck by the omission, had corrected it by a belated and supernaturally bungled paste on. This first body impresses us as crafty but dispensable, the stuff of "images": formative, but not strictly necessary for the continuation of our lives. Valéry's second body is made up of the consciousness of our inner workings. Of this one there is little to say, since most of us trudge on unaware of whether we have one or two kidneys, and only by confronting it with challenging rigors, as do mystics, does it come into prominence. The third body may be defined as body-object-of-scientific-inquiry. Valéry is complacent about it for the reason that he can see no connection between those spidery cells that scientists demonstrate in nicely colored glass slides and emotion, impulse, or artistic creativity. It should be left to professionals, he says, even though they themselves fail to understand it. Only the fourth body captures his interest. This is body-as-part-of-the-environment, indistinguishable from it, just as the small vortex that is formed in the water contained in a glass remains part of the liquid and yet is distinct from it.[4]

Poetic flights are all pardonable, but many are inaccurate. The pathologist knows that only comprehensive understanding of the third body will deliver to us the fourth one. A few years ago the scientific efforts to explain emotion and relational life seemed coarse and awkward, even to the unsophisticated. Ortega could say that it was plain how cutting off a man's head seriously interfered with his capacity to feel and think, but that, beyond this, he placed little reliance in the physiology of cerebral localizations. Today this wit is outmoded. Not that the placing of electrodes in the brain has ceased; it has gone on, ploddingly, uninterruptedly. The problem is an embarrassment of riches: research and technology begin to link together the third and the fourth bodies sooner than we anticipated. The many unseen forms of energy that surround us and affect us; the unsuspected vibrations that we emit: all are recorded in the tracings of fine sensors, in the delicate impressionism of thermography. And the conclusion is every day reinforced that if Valéry's fourth body is ever going to be revealed, the revelation will shine forth through the third one, and by no other means.

THE DEAD AS A LIVING

Y EARS performing autopsies have made me wonder what effect, if any, might have been produced by this death-related occupation upon my own personality. That trade can leave its imprint on character is an opinion of noble ancestry, for we read in the *Nicomachean Ethics* that the soldier learns courage by deliberately exposing himself to danger in battle, thus implying that virtue (as well as vice) is literally a matter of habit and "on-the-job training." As it is said jokingly that proctologists and gynecologists see the world upside down, so it may be presumed that pathologists, who see it inside out, cast an equally unbalanced, skewed, and asymmetrical glance, and this habit cannot be totally harmless. Accordingly, imputations of sullenness and pessimism to practitioners of death-related occupations are, on the surface, at least as credible as those of jollity to entertainers or callous greed to usurers. "What, in the name of heaven," goes the question most often heard, "can be expected of you, who spend your life surrounded by gloom and your working day among truculence, gore, and sadness?"

Every trade has its mystique, and at least one facet that attracts public esteem and confers glamour. In feudal times, the peasants were crushed by the most desperate abjection.

This did not bar public officials, like Sully, from declaring land tillage and cattle raising the "two breasts of France," though he never said why these "*mamelles*" suckled only the top layers of the body politic. In industrial England, menial workers lived in similar wretchedness. Yet Charles Lamb intoned the praise of chimney sweeps and attributed their aberrant appetite not to degeneration of the palate from constant inhalation of soot, but to aristocratic tendencies that lay "dormant" in the poor devils. When one poor boy became lost in the chimney passages of Arundel Castle and was found the next day, asleep on a magnificent ducal bed, Lamb had the gall to consider the incident further proof of the aristocratic descent of chimney sweeps: he could have collapsed on the floor, says Lamb, but a "mysterious instinct" led him to the bed of his ancestors! All this shows that, however hypocritical, official accolade has not been withheld from lawful occupations, even the most menial. Useful and necessary jobs are paid, if not with just remuneration, punctually with sanctimonious lip service. But the public mind has always made exception for a particular form of employment: that which requires living among the dead. Corpse handlers, like pathologists, morticians, or embalmers, are viewed with distrust. An honest reply to the question of what one does for a living is bound to suddenly break the conviviality. At times, a shade of hostility mingles with nervous distrust, and one perceives an aggressively resistant attitude, like that of a Cambridge Fellow described by Bertrand Russell, who, obsessed with death, carried a spade with him to cut the worms he saw on the lawns, and did so saying: "Yah! You haven't got me yet!" Nor is this distrust found solely among the laity. Richard Selzer, the surgeon-writer, called the pathologist "the weevil in the flour sac of Medicine" and in a humoristic essay described him as a despicable creature vilified by his interest in the morbid, depraved by prolonged exposure to evisceration and dismemberment. Against this background, I wish to maintain that such activities, as performed by pathologists, are most salutary for the character of these practitioners and lack not in ennobling and even poetic qualities.

Above all, it is of interest to note that the pathologist is among the very few who are interested in the dead *qua* dead, in a uniquely concrete way. Such a frontal and unambiguous approach is taken by no one else, not even by those who, as clergymen, scientists, mystics, or poets, might be expected to include thanatology as part of their curriculum. Except for the pathologist, those who approach the dead do so by depersonalizing them, by ceasing to see them as human beings. Divested of any individuality, the dead become contemplable.

An illustration of this poetic sidestepping is furnished by Eça de Queiros. In his essay "On the Dead," cadavers are regarded collectively and *in abstracto*. Whether they perished consumed by fevers or by cancerous growths, they were buried and later disintegrated inside the earth. Their flesh slowly rotted and melted, and the liquid products became organic juice. Sucked by the roots of plants, their substance climbed toward the sun, transformed into fruit, leaf, or flower. Those who drowned at sea were also transformed, slowly deliquescing amidst shells and corals and sand. Eventually, they came back, in the ebb and flow of tides, indistinguishable from the whiteness of spume. And even those eventually crumbled who were killed in the mountains and devoured by wild beasts or murdered in cities and left to rot in back alleys. Liquefied by bacterial enzymes, dissolved in the sun, turned into small molecules, then atoms, they were scattered as mist in the wind. The poet contrasts the well-ordered, peaceful condition of the dead with the disconsolate, nervous, and hungry condition of the living, forced to struggle to adapt to perpetually changing conditions. Eça de Queiros thus writes that "the dead are happy because they are far from the human form," interlocked in the chain of nature's transmutations, without concern for misery and decay. The scientist's abstraction is not much different, since, in his scheme, the weakness of the human condition is sighted from the perfect, pure, immaculate vantage point of organic compounds or thermodynamic reactions. In a way, scientist and poet would agree that "the perfect good is attained only by ceasing to be human."

But of these abstractions the pathologist wants no part. As soon as the dead cease to be human, they no longer interest him. In fact, he looks at life from the vantage point of the deceased. His task is to "explain" the living being by examination of the corpse: like the fool of Lucretius, he wishes to advance by backward leaps, which is what he does when he keeps "referring" his findings to the symptoms. In his constant effort to guess the faulty construction by looking at the heap of rubble, the pathologist often strikes us as unreasoning; paraphrasing Berkeley, one might say that his trade renders him "wont to infer consequences from consequences—and never the wiser for it." The temptation is great to ridicule a form of reasoning that insists on inferring causality from irreversible, terminal effects. But let those who would scoff at it consider the illustrious record of this method, and their ironies are silenced: one does not argue with success. The long and continued list of contributions of pathologic anatomy to medicine, stands as proof—a fact not researched enough by epistemologists—that, in conducting inquiries, it often pays to bridle the horse by the tail.

Consider now the plight of the pathologist. When the time for confronting the dead arrives, he stands alone: the relatives are kept in durance by grief, whence the clergy strives to free them; scientist and poet absconded, as soon as the door of the morgue was shut, through the postern of abstraction. But to the pathologist there is no escape. His task is squarely to confront the dead and, violating their most intimate individuality, to collect the information with which truthful, testable abstractions may be built. But before second-order ideas and hypotheses are constructed, he must dip his hands in blood and viscous secretions and experience revolting sensations, nauseating odors, revolting sights. In the heroic era of the science of pathology, devoted scientists thought nothing of tasting organ secretions: Giovanni Battista Morgagni, one of the founding fathers of this discipline, recorded for posterity the taste of the fluid found in splenic cysts of pigs; his disciple Valsalva did not hesitate in tasting the fluid of ovarian and renal cysts. Need we say that their present-day successors should be thankful that scientific progress has removed the need for bravery from chemical investigation? And yet, putrid exudates must still be collected, and necrotic tumors handled and weighed and sampled. As in the past, contemporary physicians must engage in the practices that Quevedo ridiculed in his "Dream of Death": they must "ask piss what they don't know. . . . And as if the urinal was going to speak to them in whispers, they approach it of their ears, till their beards are bedewed by its moisture." The anatomical concept of disease has long consolidated, but its cultivation still requires as much conviction and scientific zeal as stomach.

Perhaps in no other area is this more true than in the field of forensic pathology. Lest my indignant colleagues lash at me for dwelling on the purely subsidiary and external trappings of their occupation, I hasten to add that theirs is as venerable a scientific discipline as any other. There would be much to say of the proud record of forensic pathology as a science. The investigation of poisoning, for example, extends from the naive efforts of Chinese coroners who used to test for poisons by placing a fistful of rice in the cadaver's mouth, then feeding it to chickens to observe untoward effects, to present-day use of the most sophisticated technics, such as high-pressure liquid chromatography, to ascertain the presence of toxic substances in bodily fluids. There would even be much to say of the moral contribution of this science, since an essential part of its business is to gather evidence to be used in court, thus contributing to uphold the rule of justice in human transactions. But our concern here is exclusively with externals rather than essentials. And to the forensic pathologist, the outward structure of death is usually the horrid effect of violence on the frailty of the human body. The field of study is men, women, and children cut into small bits, bludgeoned into amorphous, bloody tatters, carbonized by high temperatures, immersed in tanks of corrosive acids, bloated by prolonged immersion in water, half eaten by rats, tunneled by maggots, skinned by abrasives, blue from asphyxia, cherry red from carbon monoxide, inconspicuously pierced with ice picks, or blown into irrecoverable shreds by industrial explosions. I confess to lacking the mettle requisite for looking beyond these externals into legal, moral, and scientific considerations. Yet one aspect of these externals I find fascinating, and it is a central preoccupation of the forensic pathologist. This is the systematic study of the formalism of death, the careful canvassing of posture, gesture, and all extrinsic circumstances that surround individual deaths.

The ways of entering into this world are limited, but those of leaving it seem infinite. This observation caught the public's attention in bygone days, and biographers took pains to note the motions of the absconding. Thus of Warren Hastings, Julius Caesar, and Pompey it is said that each veiled his face at the last moment. Socrates did the same: he covered his face, and when his friend Crito uncovered him, he was gone. The occasion was supposed to be momentous, so those with the power to solemnize it tried their best at ornamenting their exitus. Charles V of Spain, at the Yuste monastery, even hit upon the extraordinary idea of rehearsing his own funeral,

OUACHITA TECHNICAL COLLEGE

complete with tearful attendants, chapel hung in black, huge catafalque, and himself as spectator during the service. Others, afraid that dress rehearsals might not preclude surprises on opening day, made final dispositions to cover contingencies. The duke of Montmorency, suspected of habitual incest with his daughters, insisted nonetheless that his body should be clad in the raiment of a Capuchin monk. And it was well that he should have taken pains at this, says his biographer, for "without disguise he stood no chance of entering into the kingdom of heaven." As times became less religious, however, this strict attention to terminal details was pronounced to be useless. Furthermore, the external circumstances of death seemed utterly devoid of scientific meaning. A whole science, obstetrics, concerned itself with the mechanics of the arrival, whereas the mechanics of the departure were not considered a proper field of inquiry. But, lo and behold! through the efforts of forensic pathologists, the externals of death become once more a creditable field of knowledge. The moment of death is restored to scientific respectability. Whether the window was open or shut; whether the left or the right hand was raised; whether, the moment death came, the deceased looked right or left—all of these become matters of weighty importance. Whether President Kennedy's head inclined forward the moment he fell stricken by one, two, or three bullets, or whether Fred Hamptom, deputy chairman of the Black Panther Party, lay supine, prone, or semirecumbent when visited by analogous death—these become the focus of attention for historians, questions upon which all the resources of modern science are brought to bear.

From the foregoing it should be apparent that the performance of autopsies as a trade represents a unique form of human activity: unique in receiving society's distrust as usual guerdon; unique in its concrete, unambiguous confrontation with the dead; unique in its interest in the dead as dead persons, rather than abstractions. It remains yet to show how the habitual engagement in activities apparently so disagreeable, carried out in surroundings that are generally oppressive, can become an edifying experience; or how such a dark, frowned-upon occupation can contribute to the betterment of its practitioners. It is my contention that such happy consequences result from the singularly forceful way in which the autopsy teaches the double lesson of individuality and commonality in human beings.

Milton Helpern, the chief medical examiner of New York City, who personally performed tens of thousands of autopsies in his long career, reflected upon the fact that individuality stamps its mark on every part of the anatomy: no two hearts are entirely alike; the shapes of livers are never quite the same; branching vessels always ramify in a unique way. Refinements in technology only magnify individual distinctions: from a fragment of mandible or a tooth it is possible to deduce the race, age, and sex of the deceased. Today we know that bodily secretions, a hair, a bloodstain, bear the mark of the individual and that insight into the molecular arrangement of bodily parts further reveals "fingerprints" inside an ever diversifying individuality. We are thus entitled to feel special, irreplaceable, thoroughly unique. But this feeling, by itself, is unwarranted and pernicious. Constant affirmation of individual differences creates the illusion that a deep chasm cuts between the self and others. We gratify our ego by asserting most emphatically the comparisons that show ourselves in a favorable light, and, by degrees, we delude ourselves into believing that intelligence, social caste, or beauty stand between two human beings as a gulf wider than the gap between species. This is what Schopenhauer meant in stating that the "principle of individuation" is the root of conceit.

No one who has spent his life by the autopsy table is ready to believe with Hume that "nature meant original distinctions betwixt breeds of men." The fallacy that a mystical quality exalts a human being over his peers is shattered more violently by daily contemplation of our inner frailties than by any amount of theological discourse. Bishop Belzunce, during the great plague of Marseilles, declared that "God would not afflict His flock to the point of condemning the pastor," thus voicing less trust in the Almighty than confidence in a hierarchical order capable of giving him special status. Henri Martin, a philosopher of the Enlightenment, in a fit of patriotic enthusiasm wrote that, in contrast to Germans, Frenchmen exhibited a more capacious thorax with a smaller volume in the abdomen to contain the intestines. In contrast, the surgeons who examined the remains of Louis XV were amazed by the enormous length of the royal bowel and attributed it, perhaps correctly, to the rarely contravened appetite of the deceased. The glory of the Gallic race thus needed a different explanation. By the same token, the German philosophers who championed the advent of National Socialism wasted torrents of ink trying to demonstrate the superior physical powers of the Aryan, "that Prometheus of mankind, from whose shining brow the divine spark of genius has at all times flashed forth." It is perhaps not overly optimistic to suppose that, had they any familiarity with what may be found behind that shining brow (as was being deftly exposed every day in the autopsy rooms of each *Stadtkrankenhaus*), their enthusiasm for the immortal virtues of the Aryan race might have been tempered. Admittedly, this expectation is purely hypothetical, but it draws support from mental habits that grow well in the morgue. Thus the hero-worshipper tells us that Napoleon's moments of abstraction during his exile were due to intent communion with the demiurge of France's immortality. To those utterly familiar with his autopsy report, dyspepsia seems a much more likely explanation.

The conclusion is not that the practice of postmortem studies turns pathologists into benevolent propounders of the brotherhood of man or into skeptic philosophers. Any humanistic endeavor that opens up new intellectual vistas removes the instructed from the petty rancors and routine aggravations of daily life and, by doing so, may be said to exert a salutary influence upon the disposition of its pursuers. But the difference between most intellectual activities and "morbid anatomy" amounts to the difference between the abstract and the concrete. Bergson said that it is possible to gain much information about the city of Paris by reading narratives of travel and descriptions of buildings, by examining maps and studying its photographs. The student may thus come to know the exact weight of the statue of Joan of Arc or the precise distance between famous monuments. However, this knowledge cannot be compared with the knowledge provided by a ten-minute walk along the shaded Parisian boulevards, full of the sight and sounds of the renowned city. And so it is with the autopsy: its didactic impact lies entirely within its coercive power. Left to abstractions, our mind would fain seek refuge in philosophies that uphold our uniqueness, but the autopsy, in a most brutal way, reveals our sameness. We should wish to take solace in thoughts that flatter our desire for permanence when the autopsy drags us, by the hair, into the spectacle of our own dissolution.

REFLECTIONS ON
CHILD ABUSE

As a pathologist-in-training in the 1960s, my first confrontation with child abuse was a harrowing experience that took place in the atmosphere of a sleuthlike investigation. At the center was a lovely three-year-old girl, brought nearly dead to the hospital by her mother, who reported having fallen downstairs while carrying the child in her arms. The child's cherubic appearance precluded any accusation of gross neglect. The parents were in their thirties: he, a skilled technician who held a well-paid job; she, a staid housewife with many friends ready to vouch for her impeccable character. Nevertheless, the autopsy uncovered incriminating evidence that led authorities to prosecute, then to convict, the abusing parents. The lesions found were incompatible with the accident alleged to have caused them, and of which the mother bore no marks. At that time, the radiologic and pathologic appearances of willfully inflicted trauma on young children had been known for more than a decade. Yet no amount of foreknowledge and no amount of inurement to the unpleasant side of anatomic studies could have prepared us for the harrowing story told by that mangled, innocent body. Fractures in different stages of evolution bespoke repeated episodes of violence; avulsions of limb cartilages and tears of periosteum and ligaments indicated former brutal tugs on those tender limbs; galea hemorrhages, underlying neatly delineated contusions hidden by scalp hair, pointed at the furious impact of a blunt instrument—a hairbrush, as later confessed by the aggressor—against that angelic head. We were to find out subsequently that cases like this, with all its shocking horror, are common in forensic circles. Pathologists observe innumerable, nightmarish patterns of violence against children: burns on palms, soles, and buttocks of those seated in tubs of hot water; looped skin marks left by flogging with electric wire; geometrically shaped bruises inflicted by belt buckles; generalized lesions of marasmus in those killed by starvation and neglect; and, as one of many bizarre consequences of parental sadism, chemical pneumonia when soap was aspirated by a child whose mouth was forcefully "washed" or when, in one reported case,[1] pepper was used instead as punishment for unwanted utterances!

The enormity of these crimes, their senselessness, their frightening frequency—more than twenty-six thousand in New York City alone, from January to December of 1975, serious enough to be reported[2]—overwhelmed me then and crushes me today with most grievous, undiminished poignancy. On the day of that first confrontation I heard from fellow residents, virtually all foreigners, that this was a uniquely American phenomenon, that none recollected instances of such monstrous behavior in their homeland. A self-recriminatory national press seemed to echo that belief. In desperation, I nourished the naive hope that other, less violent societies held the key to a universally more humane treatment of children. But where to look? England has too shady a tradition of institutionalized abuse, as can be gleaned from the tarnished record of its famous boarding schools, which are but a natural outgrowth of society. And so do virtually all countries that descend from, or align themselves with, Anglo-Saxon tradition. In New Zealand, for instance, Section 59 of the Crimes Act states: "Domestic discipline. I. Every parent or person in place of a parent and every schoolmaster is justified in using force by way of correction towards any child or pupil under his care, if the force used is reasonable under the circumstances." And, after a paragraph, "II. The reasonableness of the force used is a question of fact." It takes no extraordinary powers of insight in human affairs to realize that delegation of such discretionary "powers of discipline" into the hands of adults seldom works to the benefit of children, an interpretation voiced by New Zealand scholars with expertise in child rearing.[3] Scandinavia, perhaps? The Scandinavian countries have much to teach the rest of the world. It is a matter of record that Scandinavian citizens have engaged in collective violence to a much lesser extent than others and that they have less to fear from the coercive power of the state (and more to be thankful for in its enlightened policies) than citizens of many other countries today. As far back as the 1920s, Sweden had statutes that prohibited corporal punishment in the secondary school. But all cannot be right in societies burdened with the highest incidence of suicide in the world and where conspicuous, semisuicidal alcoholism, a proverbial scourge, is both symptom and cause of individual alienation. Nor can this be dismissed lightly when in Finland, as an example, 68 percent of homicides and 65 percent of aggravated assaults (some, no doubt, on children) are committed under the influence of alcohol or other drugs.[4] And if such is the spectacle in countries justly renowned for advanced legislation and social progress, we might as well forsake looking into destitute and war-torn nations, where suffering is commonplace and collective feelings of compassion must daily be excepted for the sake of survival.

Should we look further, say, to the Orient? Westerners

naturally expect that the people of China, who for thousands of years have continually inhabited a densely populated region of the world, should have developed an elaborate set of rules for peaceful coexistence among neighbors. To a large extent this is true, but when it comes to the relationship between parents and children, the West expects a greater lesson, considering the extraordinary emphasis that the Chinese have placed on the virtue of filial piety from time immemorial. As a longtime student of elementary Chinese (a folly against which I now warn all who have reached the age of reason free from masochistic cravings), I am well acquainted with the material that all schoolchildren memorize in the Chinese-speaking world. These are stories that glorify children's devotion to their parents in an infinite number of settings: the child who offered himself for sacrifice in place of his condemned father and thus moved the emperor to commute the sentence; the children who sold themselves into slavery in order to raise money to build their father's tomb; the daughter who shielded her parents from an attacking tiger and confounded the beast into retreat; Wu Meng, the son who, to prevent mosquitoes from harassing his elderly parents in the summer, took off his clothes and lay down near their bed, thus attracting the mosquitoes to his own body; the little orphan boy who, abused by his stepmother when he could not bring the fish that she desired because the river was frozen, lay crying on his natural mother's tomb and, in recompense for this filial devotion, was rewarded by heaven with the miraculous emergence of a fish from the tomb, thus safeguarding him from further mistreatment; and so on. The educational goal of these narratives seems alien to the 1959 United Nations Declaration of the Rights of the Child, which says that "mankind owes to the child the best it has to give." Rather, it appears that the child's welfare comes a distant second to the parents' welfare. It might be objected that the sociocultural values of the Chinese must not be judged from a Western vantage point and that the system of filial piety works well in China because it ensures the care of the elderly. Adults who live in a society where everyone expects that children will become the main, if not the exclusive, support of their old age keenly realize that today's benevolence guarantees future welfare. Moreover, if filial piety is a virtue, the more of it the better. And is not inculcating such sound principles in the young giving them "the best that mankind has to give"?

Serious pitfalls are apparent in the Chinese system. The first one is of a general kind: unquestioning submissiveness to paternal authority, even beyond childhood, has the effects that all habitual, unreasoned acceptance of received opinion inevitably exerts; that is, it makes people's minds rigid, willing to subordinate reason to the demands of those in power, and utterly impervious to good counsel. Indeed, some scholars contend that authoritarian governments find it easier to exercise despotic rule in Chinese societies through emphasis on "filiality," which they brazenly exploit for sociopolitical ends.[5] When children's filial duty is to stoically suffer all kinds of parental punishment, it is a thin line that separates parental good judgment from dangerous abuse. A story attributed to a disciple of Confucius concludes with the moral that a son may refuse to submit to punishment if his life is endangered: not to submit would be wrong, but to let oneself be punished to death by one's father would be unfilial (presumably because the father would be left heirless). The philosopher concludes the story with Chinese directness, asking, "Which is worse? You tell me." However, the message is unrealistic and ambivalent: the offspring are accustomed to be unquestioning most of the time yet are expected to exert good judgment some of the time. A Chinese anthropologist, David Wu, puts it in more colorful terms: "It is clear that according to Confucian logic, a son should use his judgement in voluntarily submitting himself to his father's beating. He should run for his life when the stick is large enough to kill him. What if the son makes the wrong decision? He should be either an unfilial son or dead."[6] I feel tempted to add: Which is worse? You tell me.

This system leads to discrimination against women and selective abuse of girls. Elderly parents know that help is likelier to come from sons than from daughters, for the latter marry and leave the household. Therefore, to spend too much effort in cultivating the personal development of a girl would be, as a Chinese said in an interview, "like watering someone else's garden." These remarks should not be construed as implying that Chinese parents act from purely selfish motives, always expecting repayment for their care. Parents in China can be as generous and self-sacrificing as parents anywhere in the world. But even ardently patriotic Chinese would agree that to be born a girl in a traditional Chinese family "is not quite the same" as being a boy. History shows that in times of excruciating economic hardship, girls were the first to be sacrificed—often sold as slaves, concubines, or prostitutes.[7] And this tragedy, though reduced in scope, has not entirely disappeared; in Taiwan, girls of economically disadvantaged families continue to be given up for "adoption" by the well-to-do. On the authority of Wu, we know that there were between 125,000 and 180,000 "adoptive maids" in Taiwan in the 1950s and that legislation was enacted in the 1970s to protect them, thereby acknowledging the persistence of the problem. Against claims of a hypocritical middle class that the lot of these girls is not as bad as it is made to appear, there stands demographic evidence of higher mortality, very likely due to neglect, among "adopted," versus natural, daughters. Occasionally, if their fate has made them fall in the midst of a less benevolent family—and who can tell the abstruse astrology that controls Chinese fates?—these poor girls will become news items in the crime section of the *Lian he-bao* or other newspapers: sexually abused by the father, tortured by the mother, and, sometimes, beaten to death by both.

Has the Chinese Revolution completely expunged child abuse from the mainland? I doubt it. Returning travelers speak wonders of the new order or condemn it indiscriminately. It is difficult to tell fact from ideological fancy. To the extent that the causes of these excesses are economical, I am willing to believe that enormous progress has been made. But "enormous" is a relative term, in this case referring to the shameful abjection of prerevolutionary times: child abandonment, beggars milling in the streets, hideous deformities waved in the faces of tourists to obtain alms. *Any* change in this situation meant a change for the better. Now, if I were to be told that socialist cleansing has engendered a peaceful paradise where no child ever ran terrified at the sight of a wrathful parent or custodian wielding a big bamboo stick, I would ask to be excused for my skeptical disbelief. East is East and West is West, proclaimed the Victorians. But in terms of violence and aggressiveness, I hold it as true that the American vernacular says it better: "We are all in the same boat."

India's ancient tradition of nonviolence, deeply rooted in its venerable history, is a special case. In the great Mahabharata epic, whose origins go back centuries before the birth of Christ (although it did not end until centuries later), nonviolence—*ahimsa* in Sanskrit and modern Indian languages—is declared "the supreme law," the highest ideal of the perfect man. The mere sight of the *dhotī* (loincloth) of Mahatma Gandhi compelled ferocious brigands to lay aside their weapons and to follow the teachings of this holy man. It is no secret that the United States was spared a major bloodbath because Martin Luther King, Jr., adopted the doctrines of this gaunt prophet. Thus, a nervous world, ever closer to violent self-destruction, turns its anxious glance to these ascetics and yearns to learn how to apply the principle of passive resistance to the murderous world of international politics. As in the great tympanum of the cathedral at Vézelay where the huddled races of men are represented beneath the sunrays of the Gospel, so the nations of the world crowd in anxious expectation around the millenarian subcontinent, from whose peace-loving tradition is to emerge, many contend, the only valid alternative to capitalism and communism.

This picture, unfortunately, is incomplete. Together with the model principle of *ahimsa*, Indian or South Asian societies spawned its opposite. An Indian anthropologist, Bharati, speaks of it as the "Ksattriya model," because Ksattriya, or Rajput (king's son), denotes a caste whose code of conduct does not preclude direct participation in violence.[8] The Rajput shuns vegetarianism and renunciation and indulges in precisely the opposite actions. He eats meat, drinks hard liquor, and believes these habits will increase his virility. The origins of the Ksattriya model seem no less ancient, for the hoary Vedas, canonical texts of Hinduism, shaped in remote antiquity the concept of the kingly caste. And the Mahabharata epic, where the lofty principle of *ahimsa* is saluted as the supreme command, also recognized the quasi divinity of kingly force. In the "Santi Parvan" (Book of consolation) of the Mahabharata, an account is given by the speaker, Bhisma, of the sad state of the world before the advent of kings, who brought with them security for the weak and containment of the strong, but who must learn "the art of punishment." The Ksattriya model is therefore perceived as worthy of emulation by many, but none seem to espouse it more openly than the Sikhs, a North Indian community. We are all familiar with their colorful appearance—the beard, the turban, the sword that all Sikhs carry, the long underwear of ever-prepared soldiers, the iron ring on the right wrist—all this expresses the obvious symbolism of the "warrior cult," Bharati's Ksattriya model. The ideal man is no longer the self-denying hermit: it is now the "righteous soldier," slow to rise to anger, but woe to us if his fury is once ignited! That this mentality also explains the veneration expressed toward Subhash Chandra Bose (an outright Nazi and friend of Hitler) by an important segment of Indian society is a thesis defended by Bharati.[9] This frame of mind is incompatible with the spirit of reverence for life that alone can conduce to the truly compassionate treatment of children. For men who adhere to the notion that only blood can wash the stain of a perceived affront never make good fathers, and I suspect they swell the ranks of those stern disciplinarians that, in rural India, punish their sons by hanging them by the hands with ropes suspended from the rafters.[10]

Violence toward children in India has, no doubt, extremely complex social and economic roots, as it has elsewhere. This land of mystics, however, can leave its unique hallucinating imprint on the external form of the sinister. Newborn girls were killed by drowning in water in the Punjab, but by drowning in milk in Kacch; and nowhere but in India have I heard of mothers placing opium on their breasts to kill their babies with an overdose, as they did in Kathiawad; the preferred method in Gujarat was starvation, a practice so widespread at one time that Mehta reported that no girls were found in a census conducted by the British in that area in 1805.[11] Indian philosophies extoll nonviolence, chastity, and renunciation, but the subcontinent also issued forth righteous ire, blind violence, and destruction. Whatever its sources, violence unprecedented, carnage of massive proportions, death of hundreds of thousands, if not millions, took place in that region of the world during the political troubles of partition in 1947–48. This brutal, indiscriminate annihilation of human beings vividly evokes that mythical "boat" of violence in which, willy-nilly, we all cruise, and all we can say to Indians is a despondent salutation: "Welcome aboard, brothers."

No society, not even those that most loudly proclaim their detestation of violence, is exempt from the very excesses it openly condemns. Furthermore, this has always been so. In several millennia of recorded history, only a few years have elapsed without a major armed conflict taking place somewhere. And even during those brief interludes violence of one sort or another was occurring among nations, or civil strife was taking place inside national borders. Given this background, is it a wonder that adults manifest readiness to use violence against the young? Is it surprising that two-thirds of educators, police, and clergy condone the use of force in the form of spanking by hand, and that more than 10 percent of police and clergy support the use of belts, straps, and brushes?[12] Killings, massacres, tortures, destruction of entire cities, whole nations razed to the ground, are the professed goals of those engaged in an "official" conflict. For those officially "at peace," the situation is not much more reassuring: a few years ago, government officers calculated that in New York City alone one child per week is killed by a parent or caretaker.

Contemporary historians have shown that up to the eighteenth century, the "normal" condition of children was to suffer abuse, i.e., to be treated in ways that by present standards would constitute forms of abuse reportable to the authorities.[13] History was late in uncovering this shocking fact, owing to its traditional focus on collective phenomena or on the lives of exceptional individuals whose momentous achievements influenced the course of subsequent historical events. Little attention was paid to what it meant to be a schoolboy in Renaissance Italy or a child at home in ancient Macedonia. And yet the realization that childhood is the central cause of adult experience has shifted the interest of experts to the lives of private persons and their children in past ages. Since 1973, a specialized journal, the *History of Child-hood Quarterly* (now *Journal of Psychohistory*), has been devoted entirely to this research. The published findings corroborate what has been stated before: violence has been unambiguously used as the standard way to deal with children. The rod, the ferule, the stick, emerge as the most ancient instruments of discipline. Tablets disinterred in Sumer mention a "man in charge of the whip," whose responsibility it was to strike at schoolboys on the slightest infringement of classroom discipline, and he was among the first of a long line of agents empowered to mistreat children. They were succeeded by biblical prophets who rescued mankind from the degrading excesses of polytheistic religions but found this spiritual uplifting compatible with belief in the educational value of flogging. There were physicians among them, like Luke the Evangelist, but none protested against explicit injunctions given in Scripture, such as the one that reads: "Foolishness is bound in the heart of a child, but the rod of correction shall drive it far from him" (Proverbs 22:15). Later, Rome merely changed the "rod of correction" for the giant fennel stalk, or *ferula,* with which Roman schoolmasters fashioned that inimitable tool, the ferule, for the betterment of children's minds and the strengthening of their characters. To trace the subsequent evolution of this teaching aid would be idle if it were not impossible: whips followed of every imaginable sort—the cat-o'-nine-tails is but one of them—and canes and wooden and iron rods; and ingeniously devised instruments like the "flapper," which has perforations to raise blisters; and shovels and "disciplines"; and paddles with quaint inscriptions on them, for a touch of the poetic. Schoolrooms resounded with howlings and groans, like torture chambers, to which Montaigne aptly compared them.

We need not dwell on the practices of the nineteenth century: classroom torture is bounteously described by Dickens and his contemporaries. This was the time of the Romantic movement, which brought with it the most delicate poetry and the celestial harmonies of the great symphonies. However, Beethoven was known to beat his students with a knitting needle and to punish them harshly; apparently angered by want of enthusiasm for musical learning in his pupils, he actually bit them![14] But if passionate genius may be held accountable for this irrational act, only Teutonic comprehensiveness could have driven a German schoolmaster to keep a record of the various kinds of blows that he had administered to his pupils: 911,527 strokes with the stick, 124,000 lashes with the whip, and 1,115,800 boxes on the ear.[15] Which brings us to the twentieth century. And as I write these notes in the summer of 1984, I find the daily press replete with news of child abuse, stemming both from isolated individuals and from groups in official institutions. The scandal has not yet died down of preschoolers sexually abused in a nursery in California when the 11 June 1984 issue of *Time* magazine informs us that boys from five to seventeen years of age were being systematically tortured at New Bethany School in Walterboro, South Carolina. The prosecutor released to the press sufficient information to allow me to complete this brief chronicle of the favorite educational method of all times. The boys at New Bethany were flogged; the instruments used— as is congruous with the age of the computer and the space shuttle—were plastic pipes. And for those who may choose to believe that a sensationalistic press blows isolated incidents out of proportion, there is always the professional literature: researchers quote a survey of eleven hundred couples from all social strata with young children in which it was shown that 80 percent use physical punishment, including acts that exceed in severity the "reminder pat" on the buttocks; 20 percent had hit the child with some object; and 4 percent admitted to severe and dangerous handling, including the use of a weapon and biting.[16] In still another study, one-fourth of mothers were reported to be spanking their babies before the age of six months, and one-half before the age of twelve months.[17]

Cavorting figures of plump Italian *putti* were chosen by the publishers of the *Journal of Psychohistory* as a kind of distinctive logogram. If the purpose had been not purely decorative but symbolic of the nature of the findings of the research that is reported between its covers, these cupidlike figures would be most inadequate. Instead, I would have chosen *Echo of a Scream,* by the Mexican painter Siqueiros, the powerful painting that hangs in the Museum of Modern Art in New York City and which represents the crying figure of an infant clad in a ragged, blood crimson gown, sitting forlornly in what seems to be a junkyard, apparently abandoned. Juxtaposed to this crying face, the artist rendered the infant's head anew, but this time magnified, as if he attempted to depict the reverberating echo of the child's scream. Never have I seen a more powerful representation of an infant crying: mouth wide open in the grimace of a wailing at the top of its lungs—a wail that seems the unbroken scream of the long, long line of children who have suffered abandonment, hunger, exposure, and beatings; the selfsame lament that has resounded down the ages, from ancient Asia to contemporary America; the stinging, piercing cry that reverberates in our heart like the keening of agony of an innocent victim forever caught in a mortal trap.

Violence against children may be a consistent by-product of a callous and insensitive society, but what of the abuser? There is little question that some abusers are seriously psychotic, and psychiatrists alone are qualified to classify the nature of their illness. For many others, the key to their behavior is unknown. Nevertheless, psychiatrists with experience in managing child abusers have stated:

If all the people we studied were gathered together, they would not seem much different than a group picked by stopping the first several dozen people one would meet on a downtown street . . . , a cross-section of the general population. They were from all socio-economic strata— laborers, farmers, blue-collar workers, white-collar workers, and top professional people. Some were in poverty, some were relatively wealthy, but most were in-between. They lived in large metropolitan areas, small towns, and in rural communities. Housing varied from substandard hovels to high-class suburban homes. At both extremes they could be either well kept or messy.[18]

They belonged, the report goes on to say, to all levels of educational achievement, from grammar school to postgraduate university training; they had IQs above, below, and within those of the general population; they could be religious or nonreligious; if religious, they were Catholic, Jewish, or Protestant of all denominations; they were black or white or members of other ethnic groups. They seemed, in sum, very much like the rest of us. And I believe it is accurate to say that they looked very much like the rest of us simply because they *are* like the rest of us. *But they have abused children and we have not.* Are we prepared to say that if our life history had been the same as theirs we would still have been averse to violence? Are we sure that we would *never*, under *any* circumstances, act in like manner? A background of abuse in their own childhood seems to be the only characteristic that consistently sets the abusers apart from the rest of society. That they have unrealistic expectations of "nurturing" from their children or that they tend to regard physical abuse as a way of life may be subsidiary aspects of the central, overwhelming fact that they were victimized as children, that they, too, were crushed in the mortal trap. Given that the psychiatric literature has failed to identify a clearly defined pattern of mental illness[19]—"diagnostic features," as is said in medicine—could it be that efforts at labeling the offenders as examples of various forms of deviancy are yet one more attempt at setting up an "expiatory ram" in order that we might disregard our own, barely repressed propensity to violence? Are we ready to fall back on a secure feeling of complacency and rest our unconcern on the belief that an abyss cuts between *us*, the sane, the normal, and *them*, the ill, the deviant?

It is impossible to develop, in the short space of this essay, the full implications of the possible answers to these questions. I must appeal to the benevolence of the reader and end with a vague, unscientific statement that to many will sound like a hackneyed commonplace. However, like all that is self-evident, this, too, is often forgotten and needs restatement. This is that, together with positive, creative forces, each of us harbors blind, destructive impulses barely concealed by a thin veneer of civility; that the germ of violence is laid bare in the child abuser by the sheer accident of his individual experience; that, since mere chance suffices to erode this precarious containment, it is wrong, and dangerous, to bask in the supposition that an unbridgeable gap separates us from the violent; that, in a word, to a greater degree than we like to admit, we are all potential child abusers.

Past ages did not refuse to look at our double nature frontally and without veils. The noble, elevating force of reason was worshiped in the Apollonian myths, but at the same time the ancient Greeks created a Dionysian cult as tribute to the irrational, in which they reckoned the existence of uncontrolled impulse consubstantial to our nature. Thus in orgiastic ceremonials of the winter solstice, where only women participated, the forests resounded with savage screams of invocation to the deity of unrestraint: maddened by the incessant pulsation of their drums, at night, by the light of torches, holding thyrsi and with their manes agitating in the wind, these women would quarter sacrificial animals with their bare hands or, as in the Cretan ritual, would avulse with their teeth pieces of flesh from a living bull. (Perhaps it is no coincidence that today the most frequent occasion of injury by human biting is child abuse,[20] presumably inflicted by this latter-day maenad, the child-abusing mother.) It is useless to pretend that these impulses are not a part of our nature, as many stubbornly have pretended for two thousand years. This inner pulsation is not sheer animality, since at its most destructive it retains a measure of intelligence and foresight. Seneca argued in *De ira* that animals have turbid impulses, confused agitations, violent commotions, but nothing like human rage, which is why "they suddenly shift from attack to mansuetude, one minute roaring, the next minute tamely pasturing and reposed." But the rage in the child abuser, revolting as it is, meets the criteria by which the Peripatetics sought to distinguish animal fury from human rage, or, as they said, "anger." They believed that it is often sparked not by direct provocation but by perceived possibility of future offense: "I do not want my child to grow spoiled"; or by complex feelings of identification: "He is just like me"; or by a number of other atrocious counterfeits of reason. Warped reason, reason trampled by blind impulse, but reason nonetheless. For in everything human, the Apollonian and the Dionysian will be found, at bottom, intertwined; such is the double postulation of which Baudelaire spoke with a poet's intuition: "one dragging us to the infernal, one wafting us to the divine." Nor is it wholly regrettable that men are actuated by erratic and anarchic impulses, for the same urge that leads to destruction is also the spring of all that is best in human life: enthusiasm for our projects, love, and artistic creation. Without reason, impulse may turn to negativism and destruction, but without impulse, reason would be too cold, too unliving, too ready to shackle us with unyielding, cast-iron systems in which no room is left for joy and human warmth. I therefore submit that the exclusive supremacy of reason unopposed would not mean the end to all forms of child abuse. What is needed is a certain spirit of reverence, equidistant from reason and emotion in a way that Bertrand Russell outlined in paragraphs that should be obligatory reading for anyone with authority over children:

> Reverence requires imagination and vital warmth. . . . The child is weak and superficially foolish, the teacher is strong, and in an every-day sense wiser than the child. The teacher without reverence, or the bureaucrat without reverence, easily despises the child for these outward inferiorities. He thinks it his duty to "mould" the child: in imagination he is the potter with the clay. And so he gives to the child an unnatural shape, which hardens with age, producing strains and spiritual dissatisfactions, out of which grow cruelty and envy, and the belief that others must be compelled to undergo the same distortions.
> The man who has reverence will not think it his duty to "mould" the young. He feels in all that lives, but especially in human beings, and most of all in children, something sacred, indefinable, unlimited, something individual and strangely precious, the growing principle of life, an embodied fragment of the dumb striving of the world. In the presence of a child he feels an unaccountable humility—a humility not easily defensible on any rational ground, and yet somehow nearer to wisdom than the easy self-confidence of many parents and teachers.[21]

In the nearly twenty years that have passed since my first confrontation with child abuse, research on this topic has increased at an incredible rate. Contributions have accrued from sociologists, anthropologists, psychiatrists, lawyers, social workers, statisticians, law enforcement agents, epidemiologists, and physicians in all branches of medicine. A specialized journal, *Child Abuse and Neglect,* is entirely devoted to contributions related to the field. The shelves of gigantic libraries groan under the weight of ponderous volumes that continue to be added. And as a pathologist preoccupied with "the causes of death," I cannot suppress the melancholy feeling of having learned a great unstated lesson: each death is fundamentally unexplainable, but that of children slain by their parents or custodians is, of all the others, the most abstruse. For the little girl of my first experience did not die "simply" as a result of a brain hemorrhage and a fractured skull. Behind the skull trauma was the fury (and at that time some of my colleagues were naive enough to say, the wickedness) of her mother. But behind the mother's violence, the social history subsequently revealed, was a background of alcoholism and marital discord that, when discovered, added a measure of commiseration to the universal reproof. But behind this history of frustration and maladjustment was a history of victimization of the mother, who herself had been abused by her father when she was a child. Hence, guilt was split in half, for the father, by promoting maladjustment of the aggressor-daughter, seemed to share some responsibility for her acts. But behind this truculence there were yet more miseries in the father's life, though perhaps these were too remote to influence the actions of lawyers and police officers handling her case. And behind all these miseries, there stood a violent North American society, which is but a part of a world that is, and has been from time immemorial, violent par excellence. Thus the pathologist who wishes to know "the causes of death" sees the chain of causality extended by new links, daily lengthened by research, but is never closer to "the truth," never really knows the etiology of a child's death. The pathologist must be content to look at proximate causes, must be satisfied with externals while research continues to reveal causes behind the causes in an unending chain of causality, as when a man holding a mirror looks at his own image in a set of confronting mirrors, and sees a man holding a mirror, and in this mirror the image of a man holding a mirror, and so on, in infinite repetition. So the ideal autopsy report on an abused child, the only one that would do justice to the thorough correlations demanded by a scientific spirit, would be like a narrative containing a subplot and the subplot itself developing a subplot of its own. My colleagues, I am afraid, would not take kindly to the ideal format; for to read it would be like reading one of those literary works that preceded the novel as a genre (of which I believe *Don Quixote* is the outstanding example), one in which the various characters tell complex stories apparently unrelated to the leading plot, and which the reader must sit through until the leading plot, at long last, is reestablished.

TERATOLOGY

W HAT are we to make of the monster? This is a concept that our mind simply refuses to grasp. We may have recourse to Webster's Third New International Dictionary and read: "**monster** \ 'mänztə(r), -n(t)st- \ *n* -s [ME *monstre,* fr. MF,fr.*L monstrum* evil omen, monster, monstrosity, prob. fr. *monēre* to remind, warn . . .]1 *obs* : something unnaturally marvelous : PRODIGY 2a : an animal or plant departing greatly in form or structure from the usual type of its species . . . **b** : one who shows a deviation from the normal in behavior or character. . . ." And so on. In other words, like most nominal definitions, this one disappoints us because we find the same terms, albeit dissimilarly stated, in *definiens* and *definiendum*: monster is what has monstrosity; the unnatural is what is not natural, etc. But we would like more than that: we would like to ensnare a complete monster, no less, in our carefully tended conceptual net. And it will do us no good to learn that a famous bullfighter was once known throughout the Spanish-speaking world as "the monster of Córdoba" or that Goethe, after receiving a lashing in a certain Catholic encyclopedia, was dubbed "a monster of egotism."

If we are to heed nominal definitions, our search for the monster should be squarely conducted on the field of morphology, since monstrosity is "a departure in form or structure" from what is considered normal. In the forests of morphology, pathologists should find themselves perfectly at ease and able to conduct the hunt on familiar grounds. But even here the monster is an elusive creature. If teratology as a science was set up as the conceptual network to ensnare the monstrous condition, it failed miserably. And this is because, in front of the monstrous, only three choices offer themselves to the mind: either the observation is rare but known to science; or the observation is unknown to science but possible, i.e., conformable to the existing body of knowledge, wherein the fresh sighting is received as the missing piece that fills a familiar gap; or the observation is neither known to science nor in keeping with the existing body of knowledge. In the first case, the monstrous condition does not exist. In the second case, it is equally nonexistent, since the observer does not think that the observed object partakes of the "unnaturally marvelous" quality that is required in the definition. In the third case, there is no question of teratology; the observation does not even qualify as a proper field of study. Science will assign such deviancy to the limbo of skeptical, if benign, disbelief, until the observation is repeated. But if it is repeated, it is no longer monstrous. The first person to report a sighting of the Loch Ness monster in modern times was probably committed to an institution for the mentally unfit; the first one to claim having seen a Sasquatch likely fared no better, or was, at best, derided into oblivion. But the second witness to these or other similar portents was luckier: the portent had a name; it had been classified; perhaps a hypothesis had been worked out to account for the phenomenon. But a phenomenon with an explanatory hypothesis behind it is no longer a portent: it has lost its singularity, and in so doing it has lost its monstrosity.

And yet singularity is what best characterizes the monster,

for in front of the giant or the dwarf, it is not size that bothers us; it is the sudden and unprecedented breakage of an order that heretofore we thought unviolable. Eugenio D'Ors wrote: "One is not minotaur in the same way as one is hydropic; the description of a minotaur paints a portrait that belongs to a single being—whether legendary, or historical, is irrelevant. . . . The monster is alone." Precisely so. D'Ors correctly notes that the monstrous condition is neither representative nor emblematic of anything. For such condition does not result from a particular being possessing in extraordinary degree the same qualities that are found in the world of daily experience. Ugliness we confront every day. Heaviness we are well acquainted with. Largeness is familiar to us. It is therefore not enough to say that monstrosity equals extreme ugliness or extreme size or extreme weight. For this would be like placing the monster at the head of legions of ugly beings, or large and massive ones, as if we entrusted their official representation to the one who happened to possess the greatest amount of a given, common attribute. But "the authentic monster represents no one but himself." He is no standard-bearer of an army of more or less close similes. He is the exception. Accordingly, says D'Ors, he is rather the deserter than the official standard-bearer. The monster is alone.

Might not this sense of solitude, of irredeemable loneliness, be the cause of that sadness that we feel upon the sight of the deformed? For to see a malformed human being may fill us with uneasiness, or fright, but first of all oppresses us with an invincible despondency, an intolerable heaviness of heart that must be overcome before it gives way to intellectual curiosity, awe, or hostile prejudice. The ancients perhaps understood that a monster ceases to be one when it is "mass produced," when its attributes become common and shared. Therefore, as soon as they observed an isolated deviant, instantly their imagination fabricated others like it. The science of teratology lends credibility to the most fantastic accounts of ancient writers. In spite of the irate denials of more modern observers, there *are* human beings with one eye in the forehead, without nose, or with "flippers" in place of limbs. Any experienced pathologist today knows of the existence of children born covered by a scaly integument, which upon simple inspection resembles that of fish; of double-headed, four-limbed creatures; of mouthless individuals. What is remarkable is not the qualitative nature of the descriptions of ancient writers, for certainly they could have had real, living creatures as models. What is astounding is that early observers should have populated vast regions of the earth with such creatures. According to Strabo (*Geographicorum*, bk. 2), a whole race of men without mouths (astomia) lived in an area of India. Pliny, in his *Natural History* (bk. 7, chap. 2), reports them as dwellers of an area close to the source of the Ganges. And Solinus's narratives (*Polystoria*, chap. 52) further enrich the original descriptions with all manner of detail: they are a hirsute race; not having mouths, they live by respiration, and odors are to them what food is to us; too pungent an odor could kill them, which physiological peculiarity, I might add parenthetically, seems to have ruled out their ever visiting onion- and garlic-loving Mediterranean shores. Ctesias spoke of a race of Negroes with what in modern technical parlance would be called imperforate anus. Because of their organic inability to expel the solid residues of what they ingested, they had to be most careful of what they ate. Their diet, understandably, consisted mainly of fluids. They drank milk but took certain sweet roots that prevented its curdling inside the stomach. They also knew of plants that made them vomit, thus eliminating all superfluity. They were also inhabitants of remote corners of India. Tailed people lived nearby, according to Pliny (*Natural History*, bk. 7, chap. 23), but if we believe other chroniclers, a tail was no hindrance to demographic growth. Thus Pausanias affirmed that this was the normal bodily conformation of the inhabitants of certain islands (Satirid Islands); much later, Marco Polo said the same thing of a people established in Asia (*Travels*, chap. 156). In the seventeenth century, a Dutch navigator, H. J. Otto Helbiguis, affirmed that the inhabitants of the mountains of the province of Kelang, or Quelang, on the island of Formosa, were all tailed. He had actually seen two "who had tails without hair, like those of pigs," and this firsthand information may have emboldened him to vouch for the existence of tailed men in other Oriental islands. Thus "anomalous races" were fabricated in the imagination. One of their number, on occasion, could be born amongst us, but the sense of danger that issues from witnessing the blatant exception to the universal law was decreased by the knowledge that it was not, in fact, an exception; that somewhere, in a conveniently remote country, and thus posing no direct threat to us, an entire population of beings had managed to survive for whom the purported deviancy was the normal condition.

Having denied the possibility of true exceptions to the universal law, the explanation of monstrous births became a secondary, and relatively unimportant question. It could well be, proposed Aristotle, that the gods were trying to tell us something. This something, added Cicero, could not be pleasant, for he believed that congenitally malformed infants presaged ill, however wholesome their advent may be considered in remote countries. On the authority of these and other eminent men, the theory that monstrous births foreshadow misfortune enjoyed considerable popularity until well into the Age of Enlightenment. But it should not be concluded that all were ready to embrace received opinion as dogma, even if it came from such awe-inspiring personalities. Fortunato Liceto, a physician born in Rapallo, Genoa, in 1577, who lectured in philosophy at Bologna, Pisa, and Padua, slyly avoided the theological question of whether God punishes men by creating a monster and very simply demonstrated that the congenitally malformed do not announce disasters to come, at least not to their relatives and neighbors. In the greatest treatise on teratology of his time, *De monstrorum causis, natura et differentiis* (1616), Liceto affirmed that he had witnessed the birth of monstrous infants without this being followed by any noticeable ill event whatsoever in the parents' household or in the district where the birth occurred. Furthermore, Liceto was acquainted with parents who before generating a monster were seriously afflicted by the cruel ill of wretched poverty; yet, after having brought a monster into the world, they were able to chase poverty away, and this very far from them, for they raised a fortune by charging high fees for admission to see their offspring!

It could also be maintained, with some semblance of credibility, that maternal impressions unfavorably alter the formation of the fetus. The maternal-fetal binomial is an intimate one, indeed. Throughout the world the belief prevailed that a pregnant woman should be surrounded by pleasant sights and sounds, a peaceful environment, lest the offspring be disturbed while vulnerable to malformation. Nor is it to be assumed that all is known about the effects that undesirable exposures of the mother may have upon the course of gestation. That smoking exerts a deleterious effect, even fetal death, is now an incontrovertible scientific fact, yet one of relatively recent acquisition. That alcohol ingested by the mother injures the developing conceptus is now abundantly demonstrated, yet the medical literature made virtually no mention of the "fetal alcohol syndrome" until two or three decades ago. That "the sins of the father are visited upon the son" should have been suspected by medicine since the time it first became a scientific discipline, yet medicine has barely begun to uncover the mechanisms whereby potentially noxious influences reach the developing fetus by the intermediary agency of the parents, and particularly via the direct maternal-fetal route. As a medical student, I remember having smiled condescendingly when I read, in an issue of the *Chinese Medical Journal,* that Chinese physicians, at that time vigorously pursuing the congruence of contemporary Western technology with traditional Oriental folk medicine, talked about "prebirth education" and devised experiments in which sensing electrodes were applied to the mother's abdomen in order to record the physiological responses of the fetus to readings of Tang poetry and the playing of tapes of Bach. I have since learned not to smile because of these experiments, but I may be excused if I still do so when reading accounts of past Western theories that propounded the direct impress on the fetus of sights and sounds perceived by the mother. Under the pontificate of Martin IV, a lady-in-waiting of the illustrious house of Orsini gave birth to a boy all covered with hair and "endowed with bear claws." At this extraordinary occurrence everyone was astonished; the pontiff himself was profoundly moved. He gave orders that every image in his mansion representing a bear should be immediately destroyed. This he did because he was convinced—whence the certainty came no chronicler tells us—that the lady had images of bears in front of her eyes at the moment of conception. The emblem of the house of Orsini is the bear, and bears are represented in many places of the palace. It may be of interest to note that a relief effigy of a bear was carved in the stucco on the ceiling of the pontiff's bedroom. No conclusions, however, may be drawn from disconnected data. The reader would do well to remember: *Honi soit qui mal y pense.*

I have before me the remarkable eight-volume work called *Storia della teratologia,* by Dr. Cesare Taruffi, professor of pathology at the University of Bologna. Today little known, this encyclopedic, one-man effort contains a wealth of information on the early investigations relative to the anatomy of various malformations and theories of their origin. In a lengthy introduction, the author apologizes for distracting the attention of serious scientists with prefatory remarks that belong in literature, theology, or other nonscientific fields of endeavor. Nonetheless, he goes on to offer passing references to the representation of monsters in ancient Indian, Egyptian, Persian, and Middle Eastern religions preceding the appearance of Christianity. Other nonscientific aspects of teratology are reviewed in great breadth, though in little depth, since the only reason for dealing at all with such topics is, we are told, "that men at one time did believe in the reality of such superstitions and figments of the imagination." Soon the author takes us on a swift guided tour of art and world religions that lasts for about one-third of the first volume. After the lengthy introduction, the whimsical flight is over, and the author sits down to the serious business of compiling the entire world's literature of case reports on various malformations. There are ponderous chapters on the objective facts that support the causative role of short umbilical cords, abnormally implanted placentae, narrow uteri, and so on, in various human malformations. The bias is highly mechanistic, as might be expected from the teratological orientation that prevailed last century. That a certain malformation could have arisen from too strong an impression on the mother's mind is an idea that the author contemptuously assigns to the rank of crass and ignorant superstition. Anatomicopathologic descriptions at the macroscopic level reach that level of fastidious detail that nineteenth-century physicians saw fit to bequeath to subsequent generations of medical men. But after going through the full eight volumes, I am left with the feeling that the only legitimate reason why one should wish to consult Professor Taruffi's painstaking encyclopedic effort today, besides an interest in the history of medicine, would be to read the enjoyable introductory chapter of the first volume—precisely that part of the work that the author prefaced with apologies and may have hesitated to include, thinking that he might earn a bad name among his colleagues for dabbling with too much emphasis in such nonmedical subjects as art and religion.

Today, research in teratology has advanced beyond the strictly anatomic, descriptive, and mechanistic orientation that it had at the time of Dr. Taruffi's compilation. The cause of malformations has begun to be examined at the level of molecular biology. There is, for the first time in history, a scientific understanding of the general plan, the "blueprint," that cells follow in elaborating their delicate surroundings, and the very building blocks of which they are made. As details of the operational mode of the genetic code are now being worked out, it no longer seems farfetched to expect future understanding of genetic malfunction. Surely, to know which genes are active in the embryo, and how they act to sprout limbs or shape eyes, will lead to insight into the step-by-step process that results in blighting of limbs, absence of eyes, or presence of malformed organs. But such detailed knowledge is very far away, even if we are sure to attain it one day. Meantime, much of our knowledge on malformations and the empirical methods in use to classify them, and to some extent treat them, rests on the long and arduous work of anatomists, pathologists, and physicians of yore, whose untiring efforts at description built the conceptual framework upon which rests the modern science of teratology. And here it seems a legitimate duty to pay homage to the Italian genius.

The men most preoccupied with beauty were the Italians of past ages, who made the Renaissance possible and forever changed the form of Western civilization. Yet those preoccupied with monstrosity were Italians, too. Liceto classified the malformations in categories that, clothed in modern terminology, could be made acceptable even today. But Liceto had benefited from the work of Aldrovandi (died 1605), a man whose intellectual curiosity and powers of organization were truly amazing. Upon his death, Aldrovandi bequeathed to his Bolognese compatriots an enormous library and so many collections of plants, fossils, anatomic preparations, rare objects, and posthumous writings that his biographer G. Fantuzzi, never ceased to admire how a single man could have accomplished so many tasks. Aldrovandi's chief work, however, is an illustrated text that should be regarded as the first treatise on comparative teratology. As is often the case for the works of original minds, his *Monstrorum historia* is not a production free from controversy. It appears that Aldrovandi not only copied examples of malformed chickens and human beings that he had actually seen, but he included fabulous beings, working from the reports of poets, or other equally untrustworthy witnesses. The result is an atlas of teratology where original observations are shown in quaint engravings, side by side with effigies of chimeras and hippogriffs. Now, credibility is always strained when scientists are asked to believe in things for which no objective evidence can be adduced, and Aldrovandi's illustrations contain plenty of such unfounded reports. However, in many cases the author is not expressing his own opinion, and before branding him a mythomaniac we would do well to give him the benefit of the doubt. He is not always conferring the same degree of reality to each one of his illustrations. As Professor Taruffi makes plain, Aldrovandi's detractors have been quick to denigrate him without reflecting that a man of his intellectual acquirements could not have been as gullible as implied in their invectives. Furthermore, his text often collates arguments for and against a given concept, as when discussing whether monstrosities arise by sheer accident or by a detectable plan of nature, without ever expressing the author's belief. That he had an eye for, or a special sense of, monstrosity may be deduced from the general plan of his work: not only was he attempting to collect examples of human and animal malformations, but he was trying to embrace the plant kingdom, and even the minerals and the skies, in his taxonomy. He believed in the possibility of systematizing every single aberration that may occur in the universe. Universal teratology! To study every faux pas, as it were, of nature.

The Italian tradition in monstrosities may have dwindled, but I suspect it is not altogether suppressed. Whenever I see some of the shocking effigies, some of the hauntingly ugly faces that appear on the screen in the motion pictures directed by Federico Fellini, I ask myself whether, in truth, an eye for deformity might not be the other side of esthetic sensibility, with which Italians are unusually gifted. I feel tempted to propose to the appropriate scientific body that Fellini be made an honorary teratologist, for he is one of those rare men who have contributed to a field by creating a new entity and not simply by cataloging those already in existence: he is teratology incarnate. And in support of my proposal I can cite precedent. This would not be the first time that an artist sneaks unnoticed into this science, through the backdoor, one might say. Taruffi states that, when he was doing his bibliographic research in preparation for his monumental history of teratology, he came across a somewhat unusual title that an eminent scientist listed in a previously published survey of teratology. The title was *Il mostruosissimo mostruo*, by one Giovanni Rinaldi, published in Venice in 1599. It appears that the first scientist-compiler succumbed to the hyperbolic attraction of the title, which I suppose could be rendered in plain English as "the monsterest of monsters," although in the translation it loses a little of that baroque surfeit that comes in words ending in *issimo*. As it turned out, Rinaldi was no teratologist; he was a poet. The title of his book was a kind of literary conceit, by which he offered his work to a lady, saying that it was so defective that it could be considered a monster. In a way, says Rinaldi, he hopes that the monstrosity of the book should be noted by the lady to whom it is dedicated, for he has seen that ladies of her quality "serve themselves of dwarfs, beings of ugly conformation and monsters, to pass the time in amusement."

That the congenitally handicapped should have been used as objects of amusement in past ages is no source of pride in the ways of our ancestors. It is a fact, nonetheless, that the upper classes displayed an appalling callousness toward human beings whose misfortune it was to be born physically defective. Charles IX of France "collected" nine dwarfs, gifts of the king of Poland and the emperor of Germany. Clearly, to hoard conspicuous human suffering in one's household was deemed a mark of the ultimate refinement. High station was shown in the ability to entertain guests by taking them on a tour of a privately owned teratology ward. In comparison with this custom, which now strikes us as unassuaged barbarism, it is true that contemporary mores are highly civilized. But it can also be maintained that a mental mechanism may have been operative that rendered our forefathers particularly insensitive to the plight of their fellow human beings. Perhaps they regarded them as *not* human beings at all. For an obscure, irrational urge impels us to interpose an abyss between us and the monstrous. This segregation ensures a margin of safety for our lives, beyond which thrives the unthinkable, the chaotic, the threateningly exceptional. It is a reflex affirmation brought about by the sight of the shockingly ill formed that says: "This is not, nor can it ever be, myself."

Literature reflects, polished mirror that it is of our inner self, this mental mechanism. Now, research in literature, it should be recalled, is to traditional psychiatry what animal experimentation is to biology and medicine, and very often more readable. And it so happens that literary research co-incides with psychiatry in showing that the monster is seen as "otherness." Nonpsychiatrist French litterateurs have published since 1975 a series of reports on "Research of the Imaginary" centered on the idea of the monster. In one of these, Henri Baudin discusses monsters in science fiction and concludes that even purely imaginary monsters derive their inherent horror and fascination from the fact that they belong in a world that is not ours: "The reader is made to experience the sudden irruption of a being that carries with him the mystery of the beyond."[1] Thus, the monster partakes of the nature of the sacred, and it is no coincidence that monstrous figures have always been made part of religions, as attested by quaint demons in medieval churches and terrifying ones in Tibetan temples. "The sacred is the absolute form of the extra-natural, an irruption of which is manifested as a monster." Baudin carries his analysis still further. A learned examination of innumerable science-fiction themes in which monsters are participants leads him to classify imaginary monstrosity in two types that represent degrees of "otherness": monster as "Altogether Different" (*le tout autre*) and monster as "Almost Identical" (*le presque semblable*). In the first case, the threat comes from colossal dimensions, non-human emotions, incomprehensible geometries, or any of a series of inexplicable attributes, such as the emission of harmful radiation or blinding light. In the second case, the horror resides in the fact that the monster could "pass" for a being of this world when, in fact, his nature is otherworldly. For instance, he has been admitted in our midst when we realize that he is an android or a robot; or, he is part-time brother and part-time alien, like *Dr. Jekyll and Mr. Hyde*; or, still, he is of this world but has been possessed by a destructive force that is alien and inimical. The examples could be multiplied by science-fiction fans, who are familiar with the numerous variations of the central theme. Writes Baudin: "In terms of bellicose aggressivity one might say that the Altogether Different is an armed foe, bristling, screaming and thrusting—whereas the Almost Identical is a spy, a concealed enemy, all the more dangerous and obsessing for that." Now, "almost" is a key word. Real or imaginary, a monster is that which we reject, which we must needs set at a distance, that with which we can never identify. And what is true for the creatures of the mind is unfortunately true for those poor creatures that inhabit the real world and to whom an important segment of society callously continues to apply the name of "monster." The historical evolution of societal views on achondroplasia, the most common form of human dwarfism, illustrates this well. In ancient times, achondroplastics were deified outright: the Egyptian god Ptah was achondroplastic, as anyone who has seen a statuette of this deity, and who has passing acquaintance with the external appearance of this disease, can corroborate. And this is no isolated case: the god Bes, with a trunk of normal proportions, but with bowed, foreshortened limbs, is afflicted with the same, or a similar, disease. But he also has a tail, and other deformities, from which it has been deduced that, like other deities in ancient religions, he symbolizes the supernatural influences that are expressed as congenital anomalies. For this much is easy to grant: a congenitally malformed being maintains a special relationship with the Great Unknown—call it demon, deity, chance, or genetic aberration, it matters little. The realization that these beings enjoy, or suffer, a special connection with the world of the incomprehensible earned them a special status in the Roman Empire, where we see them sitting by the side of Tiberius, Alexander Severus, and Mark Antony, all of whom turned to achondroplastics for advice before making serious decisions. Late in the time of the empire their position as counselors is taken away from them, and they are thrown into the arena to fight as gladiators for the amusement of the crowd; and as if this were not humiliation enough, the Middle Ages downgrades them still further, and we find them as little more than "pets" in the royal menageries. From deity to mere toy, from suprahuman station to subhuman wretchedness, the lot of the congenitally infirm in society was never to sit peacefully among the well proportioned. Save for some isolated individuals, society never willingly drew them to her bosom in an utterly natural way, free from hypocrisy of affectation. The collective voice never said to the malformed: Come, give me your clawlike hands, your bent, infirm arms, that I may raise you to my table. Sit by me, share my food, and disregard the ravings of the religious fanatic, whose offers to serve you are but perverse pleasure at self-deprecation, or the probings of the false scientist, for whom you are nothing but an object of curiosity. Rest here while I continue to seek help. Rest in the certitude that, while I live, I will not cease to look for help: *for you are my brother.*

A uniformly jaundiced view of the collective attitudes toward the congenitally deviant would be inaccurate. Sympathy and compassion do find a place, however rarely, in the human heart. When mockery and vituperation were indiscriminately flung to the maimed and the deformed, rising Christianity did much to end this wanton abuse. In book sixteen, chapter eight of *The City of God*, Saint Augustine made this revolutionary pronouncement: the monstrously deformed are still our brothers. Insofar as they are born of human parents, they are descendants from Adam and therefore deserving of all the protection and entitled to every right that is accorded to human beings. In the historical context in which this affirmation was made, it amounted to an unprecedented, courageous dissent from the prevailing pagan attitudes. The courage that this unambiguous formulation required is difficult to appreciate today. But even Saint Augustine had reservations as to how far our tolerance should extend. Development of the argument in *The City of God* proceeds this way: Firstly, we have to accept that monstrous births take place. Saint Augustine himself had seen a man with feet shaped like crescents that terminated in only one or two toes. Since this man was born to human parents, there could be no doubt that he, too, was descended from the first man, and therefore human. Secondly, travelers tell us that in remote places of the earth entire races live that exhibit these, and other more striking, bodily conformations. It is claimed that they are descendants of Noah, displaced before the flood. Now, we are not obligated to believe those tales, but, should they be proved correct, those beings would also trace their lineage to Adam, and therefore they would be human, too. However, we know that in certain jungles live nonhuman hairy apes that walk erect and exhibit a striking humanlike appearance. But we know they are animals. Therefore, it is within the realm of possibility that uninformed people, or pranksters, should wish to make us believe in the human nature of beings that are actually animals. Consequently, if those beings are descended from Adam, they are human; but it is also possible that they are animals.

Blame a fish for swimming or a bird for flying if you should wish to blame a schoolman for his quibbling. Saint Augustine, after all, was steeped to his holy crown in the pettifoggery of medieval scholasticism. That he should have ended his apology for monsters with a lawyeresque double turn is only natural.

If once again we turn to literature, we shall confirm that it is rare for societies to live in peace with monsters. Which is why they soon come to an end or, as Baudin says, they are intrinsically "unstable." The frightening appearance of the monster rarely lasts beyond the chapter in which it is introduced; thereafter the other characters learn to deal with it. Most often it is somehow divested of its threat; in some science-fiction works a neutral or even benign nature emerges from behind the frightening appearance. In any case, monstrosity is no more. What I have not found is treatment of the monster as coequal from the start. Or, rather, I have not found it in Western literature. I did come across an interesting Chinese short story remarkable for its utterly natural confrontation of monsters. We owe it to Pu Sung-ling, who wrote during the Ching dynasty. It can be summarized as follows. The merchant Hsu, a native of the Guan-Xi province, travels in a ship that is blown adrift during a storm and ends up on an island. The island is inhabited by monsters that live in caves in the rocky cliffs of the interior. Their dwellings are geometrical cells carved in the stone; they look like the clustered cells of a beehive from afar. The monsters are the fearful yè-chā, provided with protruding fangs at each corner of the mouth, eyes that shine with an eerie reddish glow at night, and voices that sound like grunts. They are prodigiously strong and nimbler than the island's deer, on which they feed after tearing them with their steely claws. The merchant is made a prisoner of the yè-chā but soon earns their confidence by teaching them how to use fire and how to cook their quarry, which they used to eat raw. In the course of the story, a female yè-chā is brought for him to wed. They have sexual union productive of three offspring, whose outer appearance is human, but who are endowed with the physical strength of monsters. There is a scene of jealousy when a female yè-chā fancies the merchant but is chased away by the monster-wife. Later, Hsu manages to return to China, accompanied by one of his sons. This one is admitted to the imperial army, since his external appearance is human and he has learned to speak the Chinese language. Because to human appearance he joins monstrous ferocity and strength, he is enormously successful in his military career. He rises in the ranks to the position of a high officer. Years later, another merchant lands on the mysterious island. Hsu's monster-wife and hybrid children make their way to China in the merchant's ship. The wife's monstrous demeanor at first strikes terror in the hearts of the population, but, when they realize that she is the wife of a rich merchant and the mother of a general in the imperial army, they admit the newcomer unquestioningly into their society. The general's brother is also enrolled in the army. Like his brother, he prospers under the emperor's flag. A happy ending finds the family reunited, the sons covered with honors earned in the service of the celestial emperor, the daughter a solid matron of the middle class, and the merchant and his monster-wife basking in the veneration and respect that China has always bestowed upon parents and elders.

I do not know what symbolic meaning, if any, may be attributed to this story, here considerably abbreviated. It is not an ancient one, and thus it is not likely that it represents a metaphoric description of Chinese and non-Chinese "barbarians," an interpretation that is always to be kept in mind for the productions of the traditionally xenophobic people of the Middle Kingdom. What is remarkable is the matter-of-fact, plain treatment of the monster theme. Not for a moment is there an attempt on the part of anyone to redeem the beasts, to uplift them, to destroy them, or to explain the origin of their condition. The yè-chā themselves exert no pressure, develop no plans to unveil the mystery of their human prisoner. The message is quite simple: when in monsterland do as monsters do—and vice versa. If it is true that art contributes to shape the attitudes of a people as much as it reflects their current ones, then I say we need a good many counterparts of the yè-chā story in the West. Here is a story of simple and transparent tolerance, of no-nonsense acceptance of the most shocking differences. Neither the ardent zeal of the missionary nor the blind, destructive force of the conqueror ever appear. Perhaps this is what moved Voltaire to say of the Chinese, in the opening paragraph of the chapter that he devotes to them in his *Philosophy of History*: "As soon as these people began to write, they did so sensibly."

ON MALE GENITAL ANATOMY

THIS remarkable occurrence is narrated by Jung in his *Die Struktur der Seele*. In 1906, as he visited a hospital for the insane, he saw a patient peering through a window at the sun, while strangely moving his head from side to side. The patient grabbed Jung by the arm, as if wishing to show him something. He then declared that if one stared at the sun with the eyes half-shut, it was possible to see that the sun had a phallus hanging from it, that this phallus dangled from side to side, and that this oscillation, no doubt, was the origin of the wind. Four years after this incident—the timing is important in the interpretation of what followed—a modern translation of an ancient papyrus of the Mithraic cult was published, one that contained a series of visions, liturgies, and invocations. In one of the visions it was said that in the sun can be seen a "tube" (αὐλός—the same word for a wind instrument) from which the wind blows. Every time that Jung encountered a striking, unusual phenomenon, he did not ascribe it simply to chance: his high sensitivity for everything mysterious, hieratic, suggestive, led him to conduct further researches. He then noted that this vision had also been present to artists in the Middle Ages, for they had more than once represented a kind of tube, or hose-pipe, coming down from heaven and into the abdomen or under the robe of Mary. And he further noted that this pipe issues forth from the sun in some paintings and that there is no question about its association with the perception of a rushing wind, since the Holy Ghost is conceived as a breath, or *pneuma*, descending from the sun. Thus the same vision had been present in the minds of medieval Christian artists, in initiates of the ancient cult of the Persian Mithras, and in a twentieth-century madman. Along with many other reasoned experiences, Jung concluded that there are omnipresent elements of the universal, collective mind, hidden or perceived, conscious or unconscious (or both), and eternal. These are what he called *archetypes*. The very definition of this concept is problematic and can best be done "operationally," as in the quoted example. The phallic archetype is present in the human mind as the salt is present in a solution: ready to crystallize any time that conditions are favorable; ready to be expressed in symbols, the words by which it speaks to our consciousness.

With respect to such theories I confess to harboring mixed emotions. "Humble skepticism" might be the best way to name the mixture: humble, because the intellectual stature of the pioneer investigators that have ventured into the overwhelming complexity of the human mind is no less than awe-inspiring; skepticism, because we know that they went into an uncharted sea with no other tools for tracing their bearings than their genius and intuition. But with respect to the exaltation of sexuality to the all-pervading influence that psychologists and psychiatrists allow it, I believe there is no escaping from it. In all countries, during all periods, preoccupation with the generational function and its anatomical substrata has filled a larger share of the human mind than a detached survey of Homo sapiens' bodily topography—say, by an intelligent being from another planet—would have permitted us to infer.

I did not always hold this belief. There was a time when I thought that this preoccupation, or obsession, was merely contingent; something largely cultural, perhaps reinforced by temperament, but always strongly linked to the manner of individual rearing. When, decades ago, I arrived in the United States from a Latin country in which earthy references to sexual matters have managed to ensconce themselves into the national culture, my prejudice was to believe that the Anglo-Saxon attitude was purely and simply one of exclusion. The jocular title of a contemporary comedy, *No Sex, Please, We're British*, accurately reflected—I am now embarrassed to admit, I believed then—the prevailing sentiment. After all, was this not the country founded by those austere Puritans who seem to have landed on the shores of the New World as if propelled by an icy gale of antihedonism? On the surface, myriad prohibitions seemed to confirm that all corporeal presence is regarded as improper, inconvenient, or indelicate. Notwithstanding recent slackening of former restrictions, sexual topics can still hush many a conversation; allusions must not be too blunt, or too frequent; the subject must be avoided if children are present, tiptoed around in the company of women, shunned altogether in many social circles. One must be perpetually aware of all sorts of unspoken codes that cannot be infringed without sanction. To be sure, careful modulations are imperative in *any* country, for sexual repression is worldwide. But it seemed to me that Anglo-Saxon culture had outdone all others on this score. Only two or three generations ago, American matrons are reported to have covered the legs of chairs and pianos with cloth, on the wholesome supposition that, if left uncovered, the minds of male guests might wander from piano legs to human legs in the abstract, and from human legs in the abstract to human female legs in the concrete, and from here to who knows what sinful thoughts of debauchery! Grandmothers remember that in their youth they could not say "chest of drawers" without blushing, and Scottish ladies were bathing in the sea fully clothed, as a mark of modesty, shortly before three quarters of womankind sported bikinis. When I lived in Indiana, only a few years ago, I could not have found a liquor store open on a weekend, assuming that I had looked for one. Nor did such intermittent temperance stem from public health concerns—rivers of beer and hard liquor flowed the rest of the week—but from fear of profanation of the Day of the Lord, fanned by a peculiar fundamentalism that apparently took no notice of Christ's miraculous transformation of water into wine. Now, of such a people, I thought to myself, one can expect anything, except a genuine interest in sex.

This judgment, at last I realize, was hopelessly superficial and unperceptive. For in declaring such things indecent, unmentionable, a society is not really passing an official injunction on silence. Quite the contrary: an exhortation is being sounded for every citizen to fix his gaze on the very focus of censure. The austere moralist always prefaces his admonitions in attention-riveting terms: "The pen balks at describing . . ."; "I will pass in silence what followed, for fear of offending . . ."; "And now, allow me to draw the curtains of modesty. . . ." All these preambles, all these packagings, these concentric wrappings around a mysterious center of condemnation—what can they do but enhance the electrical energy with which the proscribed object is charged? Do we really expect, after being told that we are presented with an object so powerful that it must be handled with gloves, face averted, lest it blights us out of existence by merely looking at it, like the basilisk—do we really expect that most of us will pass up the opportunity to inspect it? Every black drape thrown over the hypnotizing gem of sex with the professed intent of hiding it, becomes the dark backdrop that increases its luster. And every effort at silencing its language is an effort, conscious or unconscious, at creating new languages that will give it novel and more varied expressions. The American culture, like all the others, is overeager, and never tired, of hearing about it. Witness the enormous success of all that relates to sex: the ceaseless demands for so-called experts, physicians, psychologists, "sexologists," to speak for us and to us, to write, to communicate, to give interviews; the deluge of manuals, films, handbooks, tapes, treatises, surveys, polls, reports. Somewhere around the sixteenth century, the matter-of-fact approach to this bodily function was discarded, and the West adopted a new way, that of etching around it, of shading its contours, as if better to bring it into relief. The desire to know was not dimmed: it was increased to pathologic extremes, but it was now necessary to examine the object of preoccupation by indirect light and by the method of derivative, oblique observation.

And so it was with what Jung would call the "phallic archetype." Burst out it must, for it was like the concentrated (or, rather, overconcentrated) solute dispersed in the solvent of the psyche. But words such as "penis" could not be pronounced. Instead, indirect reference, convoluted speech, euphemism, had to be used. Centuries of oblique, slanted approach resulted in an extraordinary legacy of substitute words, whereby the thing itself is hinted at, suggested behind a veil that was meant to conceal, but that in reality enhances, the mystery of the taboo. These words can be traced from literary works of the most exalted lineage down to the street slang of contemporary cities. Well known, even to stern Victorians, was the mischievousness of Shakespeare when he makes Mercutio say: "The bawdy hand of the dial is now upon the prick of noon" and makes Pistol comment, in *Henry V*: "Pistol's cock is up, / And flashing fire will follow." But despite these licentious references of the great bard, we had to wait until the present century in order to see some scholars endeavoring to trace the evolution of words used in the English-speaking world to denote the sex organs. *The Slang of Venery* lists for the male organ six hundred different words; the number, of itself, could demolish misconceptions about the "lack of interest" evinced by peoples of Anglo-Saxon tradition. In *Mrs. Grundy: Studies in English Prudery*, Peter Fryer has taken the trouble to list some of the more striking synonyms, demotic words, euphemisms, and dysphemisms used in this connection, and he added a brave attempt at tracing the time at which these words became incorporated into the language. I list some from Fryer's scholarly work:

Aaron's rod	flute	lobster
affair	foreman	machine
arbor vitae	fornicating-engine	marrow-bone
Atheneum	fowling-piece	master tool
baby-maker	gaying-instrument	mentule
banana	genitals	middle
best leg of three	goat	middle finger
catso (from It. *cazzo*)	goose's neck	middle stump
cock	gun	mole
connecting rod	hanging-Johnny	mouse
contrivance	hermit	nag
coupling pin	holy iron	nakedness
cuckoo	horn	organ
Cupid's torch	hunter	pee-wee
dingle-dangle	instrument	peg
down-leg	it	pen
drumstick	Jack-in-the-box	pencil
fiddle-bow	jiggling-bone	pendulum
fiddle-stick	joystick	pestle
finger	kidney-wiper	phallus
flap-doodle	little finger	pistol

ploughshare	rod	tail-trimmer
plug-tail	roly-poly	tenant-in-tail
P-maker	rump-splitter	thing
pointer	(live) sausage	thingunny
poker	sex	thorn in the flesh
pony	sexing piece	tickle-tail
priap	sex's pride	tool
private property	shaft of delight	touch-trap
privities	snake	trouble-guts
privy parts	spout	unruly member
(battering-) ram	sugar-stick	water-engine
rammer	sweet-meat	womb-brush
reamer	tail	worm
rector of the females	tail-tree	wriggling pole

A psychologist might have a field day examining the function that was chosen as object of appellation: excretion, generation, vehicle of pleasure for the subject, or for the hypothetical partner, or even instrument of torture, tool for infliction of pain. Moreover, what a rich symbolism behind names connoting personification! "Nimrod" is not a mere pun on "rod" but is full of Biblical connotations, for in Genesis 10:9, we read that "he was a mighty hunter before the Lord"; and equally full of such connotations is "Old Adam," the father of the race. "Polyphemus" was used in the nineteenth century and comes to us conveying I know not what ideas of blindness and size. According to Fryer, "Jack-in-the-box" was used in 1870 on account of its rhyming with "pox," as would seem most appropriate in the preantibiotic era. "Saint Peter," says Fryer, is a designation earned by an organ that "holds the keys of heaven." And in a note taken from Eric Partridge's *Dictionary of Slang* we are informed that the male organ was called "Dr. Johnson" in England, circa 1790—

1880, "perhaps because there was no one that Dr. Johnson was not prepared to stand up to."

The least one can say of this massive lexicon is that it reflects an enthusiastic participation of the English-speaking people for everything connected with what Partridge calls "the creative act." And this takes into consideration only the relatively recent vocabulary. If we had set out to compile the recorded societal perceptions of genital anatomy in the history of the world, the Library of Congress, I am afraid, could not contain the anthology. For before Christianity, the ancients had few reasons to be secretive about these matters. The Greeks, of all the ancients, most openly celebrated the organs of "creative" function, to the extent of admitting them into their religion. Whether they did this because their admirable imagination let them reach for the stars while remaining conscious of their bodies—as classical scholars are fond of telling us—or whether, their world being so filled with lewdness, they overspilled licentiousness to heaven itself and painted even the constellations with a pornographic brush—as Christian moralists, like Chesterton, have said—need not concern us here. The fact is that adoration of conspicuously male anatomy entered into sacred ritual. In the *phallophoria*, the phallus was carried in procession through the streets. The crowd followed, young and old, men and women, advancing toward the altar in the temple of Dionysus. Young girls carried on their heads the tools of sacrifice. They brought along figs, apples, wine, and the victim, a ram. The procession chanted hymns to Palles, the gay and licentious companion of Dionysus, personification of the phallus. As the procession advanced, lewd and coarse buffooneries were exchanged with the bystanders. The entire ceremony was marked by crass, obscene jesting. And after the sacrifice, and the banquet, the procession returned more aggressive, overexcited by the wine, bolder, and more fearsome.

The feminist intelligentsia has made much of the glorification of the phallus. Feminists complain that while the male organ was being elevated on pedestals, carried in processions, and generally celebrated in apotheosis through history, female genital organs were covered with obloquy, feared as symbols of mutilation, or outright hated. Confirmation of maleness in the newly born sparked celebrations the likes of which were almost never touched off upon the sight of infantile femaleness. The codpiece of Gargantua was adorned with rubies, Persian pearls, turquoises, and a large, round emerald; for the latter, Rabelais tells us, "has an erective virtue and one very comforting to the natural member." After the nurses were through decorating the infant's Gargantuan genitals, Rabelais said the area looked "gallant, succulent, dripping, always verdant, always flourishing, always fructifying, full of temperament, full of flowers, fruits and all delights. I call upon God to be my witness if it wasn't a sight worth seeing." Now, hyperbolic praise of this kind was never given, whether in fictional or historical narrative, on account of budding womanhood. Surely there is a sort of collective attitude, never present for girls, that leads to self-confident effrontery and display in tender years, when the mind forms its ideas about the hierarchies of the body. Louis XIII of France, only four or five years old, offered his penis for visitors to kiss, instead of his hand, much to the merriment of ladies-in-waiting and the ribald joking of his courtiers. This detail has come to us from the prolix day-to-day account that his tutor felt obliged to keep. However much future modesty might submerge this behavior in later years, an organ so treated in infancy and childhood could never become the object of as much contempt, fear, and denigration as has been historically heaped on female reproductive anatomy. As late as the nineteenth century, it passed for truth in official medical circles that the uterus somehow caused hysteria. I, therefore, cannot gainsay the feminists' contention that the views of society on female reproductive anatomy have been traditionally lopsided and terribly unfair to women. (Who would dare to deny such a thing, anyway, after de Beauvoir's *Second Sex*, that most admirable and devastating *j'accuse?*) But I can, without detriment to the truth, affirm that penile glorification was not always spontaneous (behind Louis XIII's "innocent" childishness was the playful malevolence of the grandes dames of the court, who amused themselves encouraging the dauphin's behavior). Nor is it true that the history of the badge of manhood has been one of uninterrupted deference and protective cuddling. In fact, from very early on, the dark forces that nestle in the recesses of the mind, and which make us the less-than-magnanimous beings that we are, took "it" as their target.

In ancient cosmogonies, the creation of the universe starts off with genital mutilation: many are the myths that describe the violent separation of the earth and the sky as attended by castration—the big bang, for the ancients, often sounds like a big ouch. And then, consider the endless, bloody attacks: according to the Orphists (?500 B.C.), Zeus, on the advice of Nyx, makes Kronos drunk on honey, ties him to a tall oak, and gelds him straightaway. But Kronos perhaps deserved it, for he had behaved no better. His mother Gaia, angry with Ouranos because he kept their offspring under the earth, manages to produce gray adamant, makes a sickle of it, and exhorts the children to take vengeance on their father. Although Kronos is the youngest, he is the most daring: he shears off his father's genitals and flings them into the sea. From the bloody drops that fall upon Gaia are born Erinyes, Gigantes, and the nymphs called Meliai; and from the genitals tossing in the deep, a white foam (*aphros*) is formed, from which, as is well known, rose Aphrodite. Castration now takes, as it were, epidemic proportions. Of the seed of Zeus dropped on the ground, a wild bisexual being named Agdistis is born. There are two versions of what happened to him. Pausanias says that the gods feared him and cut off his male organ. There is a more elaborate second version of uncertain authorship. In this one, Liber mixes wine at the spring from which Agdistis drank. While asleep, the ends of an ingenious cord fashioned out of bristles are made into nooses. One end is slipped around his genitals; the other, around his foot. The wild being wakes up, prances about, and castrates himself. From the severed member springs a fruit tree. A daughter of the river Sangarios eats from it and conceives an infant son, Attis, who somehow manages to thwart attempts at killing him by exposure. When he grows up, he becomes a young man of superhuman beauty. Agdistis falls in love with him (the latter's erotic desire was presumably unhampered by the trauma of his past experience). Attis is about to marry a young princess when Agdistis appears and drives the whole company mad. What form of madness does he provoke? Why, the self-mutilating kind, of course. In the collective frenzy, Attis cuts his genitals off, as do other guests, including the father of the bride! "Take these, Agdistis," cries Attis, " 'twas for their sake that thou didst stir this storm of frenzied mischance."

This unfriendly disposition toward external male genitals did not disappear with the passing away of paganism. For some scholars, the castrating cosmogonies may have a biblical parallel in the story of Jacob and Esau. And when the mysterious Wrestler of Genesis (32:26) "touched the hollow of Jacob's thigh in the sinew of the hip," no one seems to know what his intentions were, but I would wager that they were hostile and that he was trying to do to Jacob what Kronos did to Ouranos, and Zeus to Kronos, and Typhon to Zeus, and so on. A reputable hypothesis, and one easy to assent to, says that a relic of this proclivity to penile butchery has come down through the mists of the remote past to the present day and that it is manifested in the form of circumcision. According to *The Universal Jewish Encyclopedia*, one-seventh of all males born in the world, including all boys in Islam, are circumcised. Jews were not the first to practice this mutilation, since it was customary among the ancient Egyptians, but it is clearly in Judaism that it became a serious ritual, a basic command of religion. God expressly commands Abraham to carry out this operation (Genesis 17:10–14), and priestly legislators, taking their cues from this episode, interpret the command as the sign of a pact between God and Abraham, and through Abraham, with all the people of Israel. In a fit of enthusiasm that cannot fail to evoke images of Attis's wedding party, Abraham is circumcised, Ishmael is circumcised, and every male in the household, down to servants and attendants, must submit to the divinely decreed surgery (Genesis 18:23–27). Since then this fundamental rite cannot be overlooked with impunity. He who does not have his sons circumcised, or is himself not circumcised before his thirtieth birthday, becomes a destroyer of the covenant, since God said to Abraham: "If any male have not the flesh of his foreskin circumcised, that person shall be cut off from his people; he has broken my covenant" (Genesis 17:14). Therefore, the observance must be respected with the unfailing punctuality demanded by religion, on the eighth day after birth. It is no excuse if that day falls on a Sabbath. Holy days, like Yom Kippur, are no excuse. Even leprosy is no excuse. About the only grounds for exception that the rabbis are willing to grant are these: no circumcision is required for the third son when two preceding sons succumbed to the operation; and the operation is not required for the male infant of a third sister if each of her two sisters lost a child to circumcision (apparently a precaution against complications in families with hemophilia). What if the child is born without a prepuce? This, too, constitutes no excuse. The *mohel* (circumciser) approaches the baby held fast by the *sandek* (godfather) and is content with letting a drop of blood fall out. What if there is complex pathology, say, duplication of the penis? Here, pathology accomplishes the impossible: it exceeds Talmudic sagacity. *The Universal Jewish Encyclopedia* informs us that this, too, has been foreseen but that Talmudic scholars have made contradictory pronouncements.

I might be blamed for having focused on the purely external appearance of this ritual and then jumping to the trite conclusion that it represents an atavistic manifestation of a castrating impulse. There is, of course, an enormous mass of research to show that several interpretations are possible, all of which transcend the apparent cruelty practiced on male genital anatomy. Not the least of these is that there may be sound medical reasons behind all this incising and bloodletting. At one time or another it has been maintained by the medical profession that there is valid justification for the performance of routine circumcision on all male newborns. The profession has claimed that it prevents phimosis (inability to retract the foreskin behind the glans); that it prevents inflammation due to accumulation of secretions; that it prevents penile cancer; and that the risk of cancer of the cervix uteri is lower in the wives of circumcised males than in those with uncircumcised husbands. It has been countered that the foreskin serves as a protection of the glans against ammoniacal excoriation when the baby is in diapers; that, later, inflammation is prevented by simple practices of hygiene; that the risk of penile cancer is too low to justify routinely circumcising all newborn males, since this procedure is not without its own risks; and that the evidence on which rests the allegation of a decreased risk of cancer of the cervix in sexual partners of circumcised males is flimsy. This is not the place to examine the controversy. What cannot be ignored is that, since a conclusive answer to these questions is still not available, the decision to perform this operation—the most common surgical procedure on males in the United States today—remains unscientific. Perhaps this case was made most elegantly by Dr. Robert P. Bolande, a distinguished American pathologist of international stature and author of numerous contributions in the field of pediatric pathology. In a special article that appeared in the prestigious *New England Journal of Medicine*, he reviewed the medical work about the therapeutic and prophylactic efficacy of this practice and with characteristic honesty entitled his paper "Ritualistic Surgery."[1] The interested reader may consult this article, of which the highest praise is that it retains a lively current interest more than fifteen years after it was written. We are here content to belie the feminist assumption of a preferential treatment of the male sex organ. Rather, it seems that no sooner has the male fetus left the protection of the maternal womb than—at least in America—hostile and punitive forces converge on his genitals. Lacking universally agreed upon reasons for its performance, circumcision becomes an "act of faith"; but since Christian families have no ritualistic, mystical, or propitiatory goals in sight, this act looks disturbingly like an assault. And may Elijah, who sits in spirit at the ceremony, forgive me for my participation in the collective aggression. As a young physician, I, too, during my internship, became a *mohel* of sorts, if the name is applicable to one who shears the foreskin of unbelievers; for shearing I did, right and left, with much surgical draping and asepsis, if not with *metzitzeh* and prayers. For this, I am sorry. If today I were urged to do it again, I would rebel and would answer, like Jeremiah, that circumcision of the heart, not the foreskin, is what men need most.

Jeremiah's meaning, though somewhat cryptic, alludes to purity of intentions. If so, we must agree that penile-mediated misfortune comes to men not from inconsequential "ritualistic surgery" at birth but from irresponsible misuse of this organ in later years. Somewhere in a Castilian classic—I think it was by Cervantes himself—one reads the legend of King Rodrigo, who, having led an intemperate life, is dragged by punitive demons into the netherworld through a crack that had abruptly formed in the ground, from where flames and sulfurous emanations burst forth. And as lizardlike demons pull him down, the quondam sinner makes it clear to the terrified witnesses of his abduction that his infernal tortures start being felt in those parts of his anatomy that had sinned the most: *"Ya me comen, ya me comen, / Por do mas pecado había"* (They now eat me, they eat me, / Where there was most sin).

Curiously, the rich English synonymy that produced "rod" and its variants was never extended to "lightning rod," but there are men for whom such a word would be suitable, because they make that part of their anatomy a lightning rod of misfortune, which attracts to them disgrace and in some cases, death itself. To a greater or lesser extent, this may be a general truth for all men: this proposition is implicit in Emerson's melancholy explanation of the power of sex. He said that the Creator, wishing to ensure the preservation of the human race, overcharged sex with passion and emotional intensity at the risk of murders, knifings, suicides, blackmails, and the sundry other calamities that have always attended it. Emerson's hypothesis, I must say, strikes me as a little strained. (Without wishing to question the designs of Providence, would not oviposition, or parthenogenesis have sufficed for the purpose?) But this problem is alien to the matter at hand, which is that some men seem to make the generational function supreme over the rest, notwithstanding pains, privations, and all manner of individual and collective woe. Their portrait

could only be made accurate by using the technic of those
artificers that fashioned the statuettes of Telesphoros. In these
figurines, discovered and illustrated by archeologists, the upper
part of the body—head, caped shoulders, arms, and trunk—
can be removed, revealing a body that consists of an erect
phallus. True symbolic representation, I must say, of some
men: behind various appearances there is nothing but an erect
phallus supported by a pair of legs.

Discussions of such personalities invariably revolve around
the likes of Don Juan and Casanova. But specimens of this
complex genus are best left unexamined at this time. Artists,
historians, and, most of all, psychiatrists have left behind a
massive prattle about what, by virtue of a complete edifice
of theory, can now be regarded as a duly suffixed field of
study: donjuanism. Besides, what was once the idea of the
seducer lies now trampled and in pieces. After the analysts
were through with him, Don Juan the seducer gave way to
Don Juan the neurotic, the conflictive, the regressed, the hater
of Woman, or the seeker after maternal warmth. A journalist
once remarked that if the original Don Juan could come back
from his grave and read the massive literature of exegesis that
his exploits have given rise to (in which psychoanalysts call
him names that range from "insecure" to "homosexual"), his
only possible face-saving comment would be a line that Zor-
rilla placed in his mouth in the quaintly kitschy *Don Juan
Tenorio*: "family cackle that never bothered me one bit." No,
our attention is better turned elsewhere, to less complex personalities, to men who, placed by hazard in a position where
they could overindulge their sexual appetite, opted to take a
dive, to the last consequences. Naturally, many can be found
among the aristocracy of olden times, come to power by a
sheer accident of birth. A worthy example is King Henry IV
of France, whom the French fondly called *le bon roi* and who

has been thought by many to personify what is best in the ebullience, the wit, the saucy joie de vivre, and the lust for which many Frenchmen have become famous.

My curiosity about the Navarrese was started, in my adolescence, by reading a popular biography in which the sexual exploits of this king were held up for the admiration of posterity with a certain ring, I suspect, of national pride in the declamations of the biographer. I then came across a second biography by Ritter, also a French author, but this one was moralistic and condemnatory. Whereas the first one had referred with sympathy to the king's philandering as the playful sporting of a Gallic satyr, the second one trembled with indignation and pronounced it *"une longue chiennerie,"* and senseless promiscuity of the vilest stamp. It was then that I discovered the admirable work of Petitot editors, a multivolume compilation of the memoirs of Henry's contemporaries and innumerable documents of the time, set in contemporary language and thus accessible to the nonprofessional historian. Being young, curious, and somewhat of a francophile, I decided to look for myself and spent long hours consulting the ponderous *Documents et mémoires pour servir à l'histoire de France.* The love life of Henry, I discovered, has much to stimulate the outrage of Victorians and the fascination of all biographers. He wrote quite explicit letters to his many mistresses. This openness, frankly, comes as a refreshing breeze compared to the stiff austerity of, say, the court of the king of Spain, the superpower of those times. So, for a time I felt that, better than Don Juan or Casanova, Henry of Navarre was the personification of unadulterated Priapus. Here we had man-as-predator, and a king to boot. And judging from the glorification of his personality during his lifetime, he must have believed it himself, at least for a while. In a commemorative medal, he is represented as Hercules, club at the shoulder and all; in another medallion dated from 1592, he holds the leash of Cerberus; in a coin struck in 1600 he is an Olympian hero, crowned with laurel. Add to this his constantly being told that he was the living, breathing image of God on earth, since the kings of France are God's appointed vicars; that he was the strongest and most magnanimous being throughout the land; that he could cure scrofula by merely laying his hands on the sick—add all this and it would be a wonder if he had not believed himself, as did a large number of his subjects, that he was also an unexampled repository of sexual energy, a conviction that must have been supported by the ease of his conquests, a fringe benefit of power. Not Romeo or Tristan, but the dark and powerful Priapus. Alas, I should have reshelved the musty volumes at that point, for behind the personality cult, what miseries are revealed by the documents of the time!

"Having gone to the stables at Tignonville, in Agen," writes Agrippa d'Aubigné (adding distinctly for what purpose: "to catch by surprise the groom's whore"), the king contracted there a "*chaudepisse*," meaning a burning on urination. And, according to L'Estoile, a priest at Saint Germain-le-Vieux said in a sermon in 1592 that the king "kept a lot of whores, but that he had been repaid by having his parts hard-heated, meaning by this that he had the illness of the pouches, as was rumored." Someone put it this way: Hercules cleaned the Augean stables in one day, but the French king who posed as Hercules was bogged down by the mud of the Agen stables at Tignonville. And he could not clean it in many years, for the king of France had, against gonorrhea, the following weapons: Hercules' club, the resplendent sword of Ivry, and the healing power that he inherited from Saint Louis (active only against scrofula)—all told, an insufficient armamentarium.

Henry's affliction was probably not syphilis, the disease that devastated so many courts of Europe. But without antibiotics, other sexually transmitted diseases could be just as serious. What kind of pathology the historian must assign will perhaps never be known. Loyseau, an army physician who examined him, mentions a "*carnosité au méat urinal près de la prostate*," raising the possibility of an excrescence, the common venereal wart. However, *carnosité* is certainly a vague term, and what it might have meant to an army physician in the sixteenth century is impossible to guess. Be that as it may, during the long marches of Henry's military campaigns, the king was sometimes obliged to dismount and allow the royal physicians to introduce long silver cannulas into the royal urethra to relieve the obstruction to urination. One day Loyseau was horrified upon finding the king's penis "swollen, cold, softish and insensitive, of which I was alarmed fearing a mortification, but this was averted by light purgation and compresses." Loyseau asked how long His Majesty had suffered these complaints. Already eight years of intermittent difficulty in urination! Thus, after much discussion, Loyseau prescribed his treatment. A long silver cannula (of his own invention), daubed with "pompholigos ointment," must be introduced daily, alternating with various preparations from the botanical pharmacopoeia that include "*trochisques blancs de rhasis*," which seems to have been zinc oxide in plantain water. "Cooling injections" of gourd juice and water were also considered then what is called today "state-of-the-art" in therapy. And so, my youthful idea of the victor of Ivry wearing shining breastplate and leading the charge of the cavalry with his sword held high, gradually receded, pushed into the background by this other vision of a recumbent sovereign, surrounded by physicians bent over him. It is night; the scene takes place in his tent. Everyone receives the flickering illumination of candles. Loyseau holds in his right hand the copulative organ that sired a race of paladins, while with his left hand he lets down a silver sound, very slowly, and pauses at the short whimpers and saccadic movements of his royal patient, whose forehead is covered with drops of sweat . . .

O appendage of maleness! Lightning rod of misfortune, antenna of bane, tower of reproduction, trunk of the tree of life, column of perpetuity, pillar of the race, tube of the rushing vital wind, conduit of excretion and hose-pipe of generation: you, too, are part of the body. At birth, your blood is shed for the sake of blind belief, which some call science and others ritual. In the vigor of maturity your tumescent pride would call itself *axis mundi*. But in the eclosion of your excesses thrives the germ of disease and pain; and in the mere unfolding of time, that of decay and dysfunction. In the end, your irrepressible urgings and your plethoric haughtiness will become growing slumber, then impotence, and then nothingness. For you, too, are part of the body.

NOTES

On Embalming

1. Until recently, no author who wrote about embalming for the general public had any firsthand experience with members of the métier. This has been corrected with the appearance of an admirable volume, a work demonstrating the highest scholarly achievement and possessing the most engrossing readability, by the distinguished pathologist Guido Majno: *The Healing Hand* (Cambridge: Harvard University Press, 1975).

2. A number of publications have dealt with abuses in the practices of the funeral industry. I acknowledge my heavy debt to the masterfully written study by Jessica Mitford, *The American Way of Death* (New York: Simon and Schuster, 1963), and to the editors of *Consumer Reports* for their highly entertaining and informative book, *Funerals: Consumers' Last Rights* (New York: W.W. Norton, 1977).

Unpeaceful Afterlife

1. Martin Luis Guzmán (born in Chihuahua, Mexico, in 1887) was a superb essayist and novelist whose work centered on Mexican politics. The story of William Benton appears in *Memorias de Pancho Villa*, 14th ed. (Mexico City: Cía. General de Ediciones, 1951) and is based on actual incidents witnessed by Guzmán. It is Villa

who speaks in the memoirs, not Guzmán, with all his rustic expressions.

Of Some Bodily Appendages

1. Guido Ceronetti, *Il silenzio del corpo* (Milan: Adelphi, 1979).
2. Vladimir Nabokov, *Nikolai Gogol* (New York: New Directions, 1944), 5–7.
3. Cyrano de Bergerac: *Voyage dans la lune* (Paris: Garnier-Flammarion, 1970).
4. The technical, medical literature on these extraordinary tumors was reviewed by me in *Extragonadal Teratomas*, Atlas of Tumor Pathology, 2d ser., fascicle 18 (Washington, D.C.: Armed Forces Institute of Pathology, 1982).
5. A more recent review of the literature on caudal appendages appeared in "Human Tails and Pseudotails," *Human Pathology* 15 (May 1984): 449–53, by A. H. Dao and M. G. Netsky. True tails, capable of spontaneous motion, have been reported twenty-three times. Surgical removal is without complications, but in one case treatment was refused because the parents earned money exhibiting their tailed child.

The Body from Outside
(With Notes on the Outside of the Inside)

1. "Plotinus, the philosopher of our times, seemed ashamed of being in the body." This is the opening sentence of Porphyry's *Life of Plotinus*, which is contained in vol. 1 of *Plotinus*, trans. A. H. Armstrong (Cambridge: Harvard University Press, 1966).
2. *Gréco ou le secret de Tolède*, by Maurice Barrès, is one of those rare literary efforts that become indispensable to understanding the work of a painter. I used the 1927 edition, augmented by a few unedited pages, published by Plon-Nourrit et Cie., Paris.
3. *Barlaam and Ioasaph* was written either by Saint John of Damascus (A.D. 676–760?) or by another monk bearing the name of John. This "readaptation" of the life of Buddha at the service of Christianity once enjoyed an immense popularity but has now

fallen into oblivion. Perhaps one of the last English translations of the complete text is that of the Reverend G. R. Woodward and H. Mattingly in *St. John Damascene: Barlaam and Ioasaph* (New York: Macmillan, 1914).

4. "Réflexions simples sur le corps" (Paul Valéry,*Œuvres*, vol. I [Paris: Gallimard, 1957], 923–36) was the modest title of the essay in which Valéry develops this idea.

Reflections on Child Abuse

1. L. Adelsen, "Homicide by Pepper," *Journal of Forensic Sciences* 9(1964): 392–95.

2. Vincent J. Fontana and Douglas J. Besharov, *The Maltreated Child: The Maltreatment Syndrome in Children—A Medical, Legal and Social Guide*, 4th ed. (Springfield, Ill.: Charles C. Thomas, 1979).

3. Jane Ritchie and James Ritchie, *Growing Up in New Zealand* (London: George Allen and Unwin, 1978).

4. L. Pulkkinen, "Finland: The Search for Alternatives to Aggression," in *Aggression in Global Perspective*, ed. Arnold P. Goldstein and Marshall H. Segall (New York: Pergamon Press, 1983), 104.

5. Richard H. Solomon, *Mao's Revolution and the Chinese Political Culture* (Berkeley and Los Angeles: University of California Press, 1971); Richard W. Wilson, *Learning to Be Chinese: The Political Socialization of Children in Taiwan* (Cambridge: MIT Press, 1970).

6. David Y. H. Wu, "Child Abuse in Taiwan," in *Child Abuse and Neglect: Cross-Cultural Perspectives*, ed. Jill E. Korbin (Berkeley and Los Angeles: University of California Press, 1981), 139–65.

7. A. Wolf, "The Women of Hai-shan: A Demographic Portrait," in *Women in Chinese Society*, ed. Margery Wolf and Roxane Witke (Stanford: Stanford University Press, 1975), 89–110.

8. A. Bharati, "India: South Asian Perspectives on Aggression," in *Aggression in Global Perspective*, ed. Goldstein and Segall, 237–60.

9. A. Bharati, "Nazi Germany, Hinduism and the Third Reich," *Quest*, 1965, no. 44.

10. A. Poffenberger, "Child Rearing and Social Structure in Rural India: Toward a Cross-Cultural Definition of Child Abuse and Neglect," in *Child Abuse*, ed. Korbin, 71–95.

11. M. H. Mehta, "A Study of the Practice of Female Infanticide among the Kanbis of Gujarat," *Journal of the Gujarat Society* 28(1966): 57–66.

12. Julius Segal and Herbert Yahraes, *A Child's Journey: Forces That Shape the Lives of Our Young* (New York: McGraw-Hill, 1978).

13. Lloyd DeMause, ed., *The History of Childhood* (New York: Harper and Row, 1974).

14. Editha Sterba and Richard Sterba, *Beethoven and His Nephew*, trans. Willard R. Trask (New York: Shocken books, 1971), 89.

15. Preserved Smith, *A History of Modern Culture*, vol. 2 (New York: Henry Holt and Co., 1934), 423.

16. Segal and Yahraes, *Child's Journey*.

17. B. M. Korsch et al., "Infant Care and Punishment: A Pilot Study," *American Journal of Public Health* 55(1965): 1880–88.

18. B. F. Steele and C. B. Pollock, "A Psychiatric Study of Parents Who Abuse Infants and Small Children," in *The Battered Child*, 2d ed., ed. C. Henry Kempe and Ray E. Helfer (Chicago: University of Chicago Press, 1974), 89–133.

19. Segal and Yahraes, *Child's Journey*.

20. Fontana and Besharov, *Maltreated Child*.

21. Bertrand Russell, *Why Men Fight: A Method of Abolishing the International Duel* (New York: Century Co., 1917).

Teratology

1. Henri Baudin, *Le monstre dans la science-fiction* (Paris: Lettres Modernes, 1976).

On Male Genital Anatomy

1. Robert P. Bolande, "Ritualistic Surgery," *New England Journal of Medicine* 280 (no. 11) (March 13, 1969): 591–96.

OUACHITA TECHNICAL COLLEGE